"You've simplified the complicated. Congratulations."
—John Miller, Miller Integrated
Health Management, Australia

"As a fellow collector of food jokes, I have a fondness for 'corn.' I like your food-humor."
—Kristen Browning-Blas, Fitness Editor/
Features Writer, *The Denver Post*

"Quinn's article on nutritional genomics...Well done!"
—Elaine Trujillo, MS, RD; National Cancer
Institute, National Institutes of Health

ALSO BY Barbara Quinn

QUINN ON NUTRITION
Nutrition Health Matters
Monterey County Herald

The Diabetes DTOUR Diet
The Diabetes DTOUR Diet Cookbook
Rodale, Inc.

QUINN-ESSENTIAL Nutrition

The Uncomplicated Science of Eating

Barbara A. Quinn, MS, RD, CDE

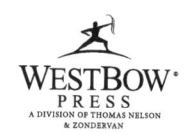

WESTBOW PRESS
A DIVISION OF THOMAS NELSON
& ZONDERVAN

Copyright © 2015 Barbara A. Quinn.

All rights reserved. No part of this book may be used or reproduced by any means, graphic, electronic, or mechanical, including photocopying, recording, taping or by any information storage retrieval system without the written permission of the publisher except in the case of brief quotations embodied in critical articles and reviews.

All photos not credited with another source are owned by Barbara Quinn

WestBow Press books may be ordered through booksellers or by contacting:

WestBow Press
A Division of Thomas Nelson & Zondervan
1663 Liberty Drive
Bloomington, IN 47403
www.westbowpress.com
1 (866) 928-1240

Because of the dynamic nature of the Internet, any web addresses or links contained in this book may have changed since publication and may no longer be valid. The views expressed in this work are solely those of the author and do not necessarily reflect the views of the publisher, and the publisher hereby disclaims any responsibility for them.

Any people depicted in stock imagery provided by Thinkstock are models, and such images are being used for illustrative purposes only.
Certain stock imagery © Thinkstock.

ISBN: 978-1-4908-7487-6 (sc)
ISBN: 978-1-4908-7485-2 (hc)
ISBN: 978-1-4908-7486-9 (e)

Library of Congress Control Number: 2015905201

Print information available on the last page.

WestBow Press rev. date: 05/20/2015

ACKNOWLEDGEMENT

To the Community Hospital of the Monterey Peninsula for supporting the birth and life of my weekly column, QUINN ON NUTRITION

To faithful readers who continue to keep me on my nutritional toes

To precious family and friends who love me even when I write stories about you. And to Michael Cook in particular, who heard my plea for a catchy title for this book, and nailed it.

To God, Who provided it all.

"Enough is as good as a feast."
~English Proverb

PREFACE

It was 1993 and a busy day at Community Hospital of the Monterey Peninsula, or what locals refer to as "CHOMP." As one of the registered dietitians on staff, I provided nutrition therapy to patients on the nursing floors, from the birth center to the intensive care unit. Between these duties, we squeezed in time to see outpatients, walk-in clients who had been referred by their doctors for nutrition counseling.

During one break in the action, I answered an incoming call. On the line was the sweet voice of Barbara Taylor, revered food writer for our local newspaper, *The Monterey County Herald*. Barbara (nice name) had a question about the nutrition content of a recipe she was planning to use in her column. I happily answered her inquiry and she thanked me. I ended our conversation with, "Let us know if we can help you with anything else."

A week later, she called back. "What did you mean by 'anything else'?" she asked.

"Oh...well," I stumbled. "We can analyze recipes for their nutrient content, or answer any nutrition questions."

And that is how it began. Over the next few weeks, I drove to Barbara's house in Pebble Beach to discuss—over tea and homemade goodies—her upcoming food topics. She asked me to write some key nutrition points which she submitted along with her column each week. Thankfully, her editor did not object. I was thrilled.

A few months later, I got a call from the features editor. "Would you be interested in writing a weekly nutrition column?" he asked.

With no idea what this commitment meant, I blurted out, "Sure!" So, on October 13, 1993, ON NUTRITION (now QUINN ON NUTRITION) made its debut in the *Food* section of the *Monterey County Herald*. My first solo column was titled, "Think Health, Not Weight." And after a painful look at my first mug shot, a more accurate title may have been, "Think again."

My hope is that after two decades, some things have changed for the better. Emerging evidence continues to warrant revised recommendations while some age-old advice remains spot on. Some topics spark controversy and passionate debate. You will find them all within these pages.

Life happens...to all of us. Memories and valuable lessons remain, however. As I wrote in 2008 at the height of gut-wrenching changes in my own life:

I'm grateful that, with proper nourishment, broken bones and broken hearts can become stronger than they ever were before. And I am thankful for friends and family who continue to provide that nourishment. You know who you are.

I am thankful for rain in summer and sunshine in winter and every circumstance that brings us life and growth. And I am thankful to God, who reminds me each new day that life is a journey; so I'd better take care of this vehicle He has provided for the trip.

INTRODUCTION

Is it true that..? Is it OK to...? What do you think about...? I get these types of questions on a daily basis from patients, clients, and friends who know what I do for a living.

Nutrition is not a simple science. Ongoing research continues to uncover the intricacies of food components and their effects on our health. Making sense of it all can be darn frustrating.

Be assured what you read here is based on solid nutrition science..within the scope of real life. Nibble on a topic or two as your appetite allows. If you struggle with your weight, if you blow your diet with every holiday, if you want to understand the latest and greatest diet fad...keep reading.

Remember too, that our understanding of food and nutrition is not static. You will therefore find a "Reflection" at the end of some sections to explain our most recent understanding of a topic.

Lastly, remember that food and eating are to be enjoyed. May you absorb a few chuckles as you ingest some corny food humor in the final chapter.

Dig in!

CONTENTS

I. Nutrition Essentials 1
    What is Normal Eating? 1
    Are You an Apple or a Pear? 3
    Cultural Eating at your Desk 4
    Timing Meals 6
    Defining Where Food Comes From 8
    Organized Econovores 10
    Food Plan for Emergencies 11
    Feeding Teeth 13
    Finding Fiber with Ted 15
    Nutrition Mixtures 17
    Farm Tour 18
    What Ranchers Do 21

II. Optimal Nutrition 23
    Secrets of Fish 23
    Benefits of Berries 25
    All 'Choked Up 27
    Prebiotics and Probiotics 29
    G is for Garlic 32
    FAQ's about Chile 34
    Herbs and Spices 36
    Spice up your Life 38
    A Dozen Facts about Nuts 40
    Soybeans and the Science of Pluto 42

III.	**Reducing the Risks**	44
	Nutrients to Boost Immunity	44
	When Good Food goes Bad	45
	Ward Off Memory Loss	47
	Cholesterol Quiz	49
	Answers about Salt	51
	Steps to Prevent Osteoporosis	53
	Can Do's to Lower Breast Cancer Risk	54
	Eat to Beat Cancer	57
	Burning Reasons Not to Smoke	58
	Formula for Bright Eyes	60
	Dirty Dozen in Perspective	63
IV.	**Nutrition Solutions**	65
	Understanding Food Allergies	65
	Diet to Ease Sore Joints	67
	Gout: Tale of the Aching Toe	69
	Diet to Fight Yeast Infections	70
	Healing Broken Bones	72
	Celiac disease and Gluten	74
	Gluten-Free Defined at Last	76
	Overcoming Bad Bugs with Good	78
	Dietary Solutions for Diverticulitis	79
	Diet-Bladder-Pain Connection	81
V.	**Weighty Issues**	83
	Think Health Not Weight	83
	What's Not True about Weight Loss Products	85
	Understanding Carbohydrates	86
	Beware the hCG diet	88
	Are you an Easy Keeper?	90
	Vitamin C Affects Weight	91
	You Can be Too Thin	93
	Will's Weight Loss Plan	95
	No Miracle in Miracle Diet	96

	100-Calorie Difference	98
	Avoid Weight Issues with Kids	99
VI.	**Diabetes Defense**	103
	Steps to Prevent Diabetes	103
	Diabetes Quiz for Life	104
	Sleep and Diabetes: What's the Connection?	106
	An Irishman Talks Diabetes	108
	Help Kids Dodge Diabetes	109
	Understanding the Glycemic Index	111
	Winning the Gold Against Type 1 Diabetes	113
VII.	**Researching the Research**	115
	Nutrition Alters Genes	115
	Coconut Oil Update	117
	Organic Junk Food	120
	Milk Thistle: Weed or Medicine?	122
	Make Whey for Dairy	124
	Is Sugar Addictive?	126
	Lowdown on Sugar Substitutes	126
	D-latest on the Sunshine Vitamin	129
	Grass Fed Beef	131
VIII.	**Confusing Controversies**	133
	Fasting and Detox Diets	133
	Nitrates and Nitrites	134
	Debating Cholesterol with Dr. Roy	136
	Cardiologist Response to Cholesterol and Coconut Oil	137
	Are Milk Drinkers Big Babies?	140
	Wheat Belly	142
	Claims And Facts About Raspberry Ketones	144
	Science of GMO's	146
	Facts about High Fructose Corn Syrup	149
	Essentials of Fluoride	151

  Dose Makes the Poison 153
  Understanding Pesticide Use 155

IX. **Nutrition for A Lifetime** 158
  Nutrition Nursery Rhymes 158
  Basic Rules for Feeding Kids…and Puppies 159
  Feeding Miss Frances 161
  Teaching kids to eat..but not too much 164
  Recipe for Graduating into Life 166
  Pep Goes to College 167
  Words for a Wise Graduate 168
  Advice for Newlyweds 169
  Life Lessons from Roy and Marge 170
  Proven Behaviors that Add Years to Life 172
  Living to 100 174

X. **Comfort Food** 176
  Why we Eat 176
  Stress Affects Nutrition 177
  Comforting Food 179
  When Friends Come to Visit 180
  Emotional Eating 182
  Chocolate: Food or Drug? 183
  To the heart of Chocolate 185
  Advice from a Horse 186

XI. **Fueling Active Bodies** 188
  Physical Therapist's Reasons to Exercise 188
  Game Plan for Nutrition 190
  Wrestling with Making Weight 192
  Touchdown: Football Nutrition 193
  Owners Manual for the Human Machine 195
  Golf Terms 197
  Eat, Sleep Swim: What Champions Do 198
  Race Regimen 200

XII.	**Eating on the Road**	204
	Road Trip Nutrition	204
	Minnesota Nice	205
	Nebraska Red	206
	Holiday Travel Diet	208
	Nutrition Mile Marker	209
	Girls in the City	211
	Rules for Flying	212
	Football Portions	214
XIII.	**Special Occasion Nutrition**	216
	Brian's Millennium Feast	216
	New Year Expectations	218
	Valentine's Surprises	220
	Grandma Quinn's Irish Soda Bread	221
	Eggs-cellent Easter	223
	Kentucky Derby Party	225
	Facts about the Great Pumpkin	227
	Tricks with Halloween Treats	229
	How to Gain Weight over the Holidays	230
	Thanksgiving a functional holiday	232
	Vintners' Holiday	233
	Cookie Exchange	234
	The Week before Christmas Poem	237
XIV.	**Eating Styles**	239
	Nutrition for One	239
	Land of Enchantment	240
	Mediterranean Diet	242
	Eating Vegetarian	245
	Families that eat Together	247
	Live to Eat or Eat to Live?	248
	Navajo Ways	250

XV.	**Readers Questions**	253
	Paleo diet	253
	Of Eggs and Grains	254
	Margarine	256
	Kids Who Don't Eat Meat	258
	3000 Pounds of Peanut Butter Later	259
	Chia and Orange Juice	260
	Mucus and Inflammation	261
	Lactose Intolerance	264
	Unfermented Soy	265
	Going for the Mold..on Cheese	266
	Iodine and Yogurt	268
	Consequences of Fiber	268
	Sugar Definitions	270
XVI.	**Men Only**	272
	Guy to Guy: You need to know This	272
	A Guy's Nutrition Advice to Girls	273
	Men's Health Quiz	275
	The 'Morel' of the Story	276
	Nutrition Lessons from Dad	278
XVII.	**Just for Women**	280
	Nutrition to prevent birth defects	280
	Pregnancy Weight Gain Guide	282
	Amazing Tru-Breast	284
	Princess Diet	285
	Managing Gestational Diabetes	287
	Recipe for Multiple Buns in the Oven	288
	Applause for Menopause	290
XVIII.	**Drink to Health**	293
	Reasons to Have a Cup of Tea	293
	Learning about caffeine	296
	Coffee Perks	299
	Benefits and Risks of Kombucha Tea	301

	Wine and the French Paradox	302
	How Alcohol Affects Nutrition	305
XIX.	**Nutrition Humor**	307
	April Fools	307
	Corny Food Jokes	308
	Doughboy and other Favorites	309
	Fun with Potatoes	310
	Proof Laughter is Good for your Health	312

NUTRITION ESSENTIALS

WHAT IS NORMAL EATING?

After working many years as a registered dietitian, it occurs to me that few folks actually know what we nutrition people do. Fortunately the image of a little old lady with a hairnet and frumpy shoes stirring a pot of soup is fading from most people's view of our profession. Not that I never wear frumpy shoes. But some misconceptions remain.

During a recent radio interview for instance, the host asked with surprise, "So you don't cook the food for the hospital?"

My mother-in-law once questioned, "You mean you write in medical charts?"

Some see nutrition professionals as diet police who wield giant carrot sticks to admonish the transgressions of nutritional heathens. In reality, my job as a clinical dietitian has little to do with food preparation (our chefs do that) and everything to do with a practice called medical nutrition therapy. I review patients' medical histories and laboratory results. I measure physical parameters and calculate nutrient goals. And yes, I write in medical charts.

How are registered dietitians (RD's) different from nutritionists?

- RD's have earned bachelors, masters, or doctoral degrees from accredited universities. We are specifically trained in the science of nutrition. (Yes, nutrition is a science.)

- We work closely with physicians to augment their patients' medical care.
- We live in the real world just like you. We enjoy eating lots of different kinds of foods; you may even find some junk food in our shopping carts on occasion. But it will be buried under the vegetables.
- We may or may not be gourmet cooks. But we appreciate that food promotes our social as well as physical well-being. So we will always be happy to come to your house for dinner.
- We believe in normal eating. For this reason you will spot us at grower's markets, pizza parlors, and seafood festivals. What is normal eating? Here is how Ellyn Satter, registered dietitian and author of *How to Get Your Kids to Eat…but Not too Much* (Bull Publishing, 1987), describes it:

"Normal eating is being able to eat when you are hungry and continue eating until you are satisfied. It is being able to choose and eat food you like.

"Normal eating is being able to use some moderate constraint on your food selection to get the right food…but not being so restrictive that you miss out on pleasurable foods.

"Normal eating is three meals a day…or it can be choosing to munch along the day. It is leaving some cookies on the plate because you know you can have some again tomorrow.

"Normal eating is over-eating at times and wishing you had eaten less. It is also under-eating at times and wishing you had more. It is trusting your body to make up for some of your mistakes in eating.

"Normal eating takes up some of your time and attention…but it keeps its place as only one important area of your life. Normal eating is flexible. It varies in response to your emotions, your schedule, your hunger and your proximity to food."

So there you have it. You can call us dietitians or you can call us nutritionists. Just don't call us too late.

Quinn-Essential Nutrition

> *REFLECTION: As of 2013, nutrition professionals may use "registered dietitian nutritionist" (RDN) in place of "registered dietitian" (RD). What still holds true is that every dietitian is a nutritionist, but not every "nutritionist" is a registered dietitian nutritionist.*

ARE YOU AN APPLE OR A PEAR?

I discovered some wild geraniums growing behind our house a few years ago. They were long and spindly...obviously malnourished and sunlight-deprived. But they were still blooming, straining for energy from the sun.

I had grand thoughts for these hearty souls as I transplanted them to sunnier spots around the house. Surely, I thought, with nurturing food and sunlight, they would soon transform into big fluffy bursts of color.

My geraniums grew all right; they flourished. But they remained long and leggy. I pruned them to encourage full growth. I fertilized them. I changed their living arrangements. They got brighter and healthier...but stayed spindly.

Was it my lack of botanical skills that kept them so stubbornly leggy? Why couldn't they look more like the fluffy marigolds in my neighbor's yard?

It made me think about our bodies. Some are naturally long and spindly; others are full and fluffy. Some reach for the sun while others stay low to the ground. Even with the best fertilizers and pruning techniques, we inherit our fundamental body types, say scientists. What we eat and how we exercise can reshape us somewhat. But our tendencies to be lean or full-sized are determined largely by our genetic codes.

People are described as "apples" or "pears," for example; and it has nothing to do with their taste for fruit. Rather these terms describe general body shapes passed on to you from your parents. (Apples tend to produce apples and pears tend to produce pears, and my family is a nice salad of apples and pears.)

We apples have waists about the same size as our hips. When apples gain weight, it tends to settle around the middle, close to our hearts. Plump apples have more risks for heart problems, diabetes, and high blood pressure, say researchers.

Pears tend to store their energy reserves (fat) below the waist, farther away from their hearts. These shapely folks have a waist substantially smaller than their hips. Pears appear to be at a lower risk for weight-related diseases than we Granny Smith's or Pippins.

Even in the best gardens of life, we can't really change the basic structure of our bodies. Still, whether we are spindly geraniums or fluffy marigolds, we need regular feeding and occasional pruning to keep us stretching toward the sun.

CULTURAL EATING AT YOUR DESK

My friend Michelle is helping me compile this book of nutrition columns. So in a recent course of conversation, she began to quiz me.

"Have you written anything on cultural eating? she asked.

I half-attentively looked up from my task.

"You know," she said. "Every culture has its favorite foods; those that are family traditions. For example, I have my mother's original recipe for a yummy Greek dish called *pastitsio*. I'm changing some of the ingredients to make it healthier."

Is it just as yummy? I asked.

"Come over some evening and we'll cook it," she said. "And have you written about eating at your desk? Eating on the run?"

I stopped to think. I've threatened my editors that I may pop in unannounced someday just to see what they munch on while they work. But I've yet to do that.

"Now that would be a good column," she said as she got up and walked across her office. "Did I show you my 'salad on the go'?" she asked excitedly as she held up a wide-mouth Mason jar layered with colorful ingredients.

I put my papers down to pay more attention.

"It's pretty simple!" she said. "I got it from my friend Angela, who got it from her friend Virginia. You need wide-mouthed, quart-size jars. I suppose you could do a pint jar, but that's not a whole meal." She smiled.

"Put the dressing (or a little olive oil and balsamic) on the bottom. Add spices if you like. Then layer the heaviest veggies–-broccoli, snow peas, artichoke hearts, mushrooms, shredded carrots.

"Next add tomatoes, crumbled feta, bacon bits (or a soy bacon substitute). Then layer sliced hard-boiled eggs and one-sixth of an avocado. Add red-leaf lettuce or whatever you prefer. And top with grilled chicken breast. I add a dollop of Greek 'of course' yogurt," she concludes. "I make four jars at a time and keep them in the refrigerator. When lunch time rolls around, I shake it up. And away I go!"

Very cool! I said as she finally had my undivided attention. It's colorful! And healthful! And...cultural. And fit for eating at your desk!

"And what about comfort food? Michelle continued as we resumed our project. "You really need to write about that."

It looks like I just did. Thanks, Michelle.

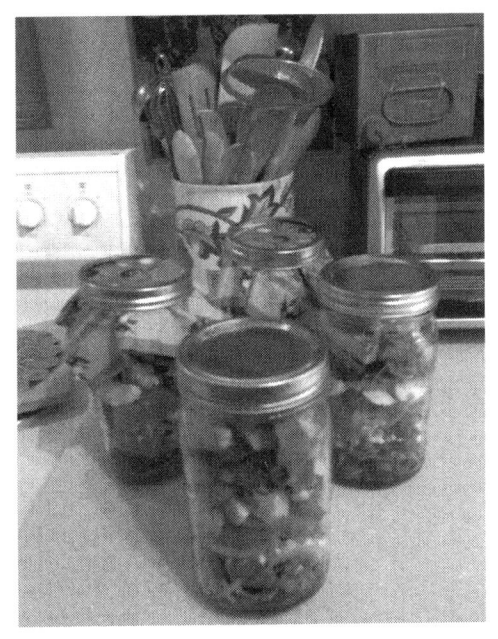

Salad on the Go
Photo credit: ©2013 Michelle Manos Design

TIMING MEALS

It's been a long day at work. We have company when we get home. The company happens to include Sally, the finest pie baker in the western United States...or at least among everyone who knows her. And there it is, a freshly baked apple pie, waiting for me on the kitchen counter. Does it affect my weight if I eat extra food, like pie, late in the day? How does the timing of my meals and snacks affect my health?

Back in my college days, I volunteered for a research project intended to answer these questions. As part of a weight loss study, we were allowed to consume 1000 calories a day. My group was further instructed to eat our allotted calories anytime before 1:00 p.m. After that time, we could only consume water. A second group of participants in this study were told to hold off eating their 1000 calories until *after* 1 p.m. each day.

The results were interesting. Even though both groups ate the same number of calories, those of us who ate earlier in the day lost more weight. This study also taught me how easy it was to go to bed on time when I couldn't stay up to eat. And it *really* made me look forward to eating breakfast.

More recent studies confirm that weight loss is generally more dramatic when people eat most of their calories earlier in the day. Interesting, however, these same studies also found that lean body tissue (muscle) is better preserved if we eat later in the day, too.

So, just for conversation, let's say I'm going to eat a large piece of apple pie. Does it matter if I eat it all at once or in three small servings over the course of the day? One study found no difference in weight between people who ate three meals a day versus one if their calorie intake was the same. However, the volunteers who ate just one meal a day reported feeling more hungry during the day. Cholesterol and glucose levels were also somewhat higher in the one-meal-a-day group.

Neither is it a good idea to nibble on pie willy nilly throughout the day. Studies show that people who eat erratically (six or more various times a day) tend to burn *fewer* calories than folks who eat meals and snacks at more regular times. Consistent meal times can curb hunger and even help our bodies to burn fat more efficiently, say experts.

Generally then, meals earlier in the day are more advantageous to my waistline than late night gorging. Now about that apple pie...

REFLECTION: Studies continue to show that eating breakfast on a regular basis makes us less likely to be overweight. Our likelihood to stay slim is also increased when most of our calories are consumed earlier rather than later in the day.

Barbara A. Quinn, MS, RD, CDE

DEFINING WHERE FOOD COMES FROM

While buying groceries, I overheard a woman ask an employee about the eggs from cage-free chickens. "How often do they get out of their cages?" she asked.

"Our chickens are as 'cage-free' as we can find," he said.

"But how free are they…really?" she continued.

"They are as cage-free as we can find," he repeated.

Because many of us don't know where our food comes from, some have lost trust in our food supply, according to food scientist Dr. Gary Smith, at a meeting on this topic at Colorado State University.

"What if we knew the story behind every food we ate?" he challenged. "Where it came from, who grew it and how? How differently would we eat if we knew the people who produced our food? Consumers deserve to know about their food to allow them to make prudent purchasing choices."

Here are some definitions that may be helpful:

"USDA Certified Organic" means the product meets federal organic standards and is produced with no synthetic fertilizers, irradiation, or genetic engineering.

"Organic" defines a product that is produced with at least 95 percent organic ingredients.

"Made with Organic Ingredients" means a product contains at least 70 percent organic ingredients.

"No hormones" means the food animal was raised without the use of hormones. By the way, this claim is not used on pork or poultry labels, since hormones have never been used in these animals.

Also note that a food labeled "organic" is not necessarily hormone-free. Hormones are proteins that carry messages to living cells, Dr. Smith explained. And minuscule amounts of naturally occurring hormones reside in everything from cabbage to milk.

A three-ounce serving of beef, for example, contains 1.3 nanograms of estrogen. (One nanogram is one-billionth of a gram.) The same amount of beef from a steer treated with a growth hormone contains 1.9 nanograms. An average adult man produces 136,000 nanograms of estrogen every day; a woman produces a million times more than that. A serving of ice cream, Smith estimates, contains 274 times more estrogen than a 3-ounce steak from an animal that received a growth hormone.

"Natural" generally means a product is minimally processed and contains no artificial ingredients or added color. This could be true of an apple or a poisonous mushroom.

"Naturally raised" is currently undefined, according to Smith.

"Antibiotic-free" defines animals that have not been treated with antibiotics. Some veterinarians argue that all cattle are virtually free of antibiotics since federal law prohibits antibiotic use in cattle within 45 days of slaughter. This gives time for the medication to be entirely cleared from the body. Also, the practice of mixing antibiotics into cattle feed as a preventive measure was stopped in 1985, according to the *National Cattleman's Beef Association*.

REFLECTION: Are antibiotics used for livestock making humans more resistant to antibiotics? Not likely, according to a recent report, "Antibiotic Resistance Threats in the United States, 2013" by the Centers for Disease Control and Prevention (CDC). The real problem is inappropriate use of antibiotics prescribed for human health, says the CDC. The report confirms that 50 percent of the antibiotics used by humans are not prescribed appropriately, which can lead to antibiotic resistance.

Is organic and antibiotic-free always better? No scientific evidence has concluded a nutritional or bacterial benefit of one over the other, says registered dietitian Keith Ayoob, Associate Clinical Professor at Albert Einstein College of Medicine. Some studies suggest our food might actually be less safe if farmers stopped using antibiotics to treat their sick animals, says Michael Doyle, PhD, Professor of Food Microbiology at the University of Georgia. What we need, say experts, is to strike the right balance.

ORGANIZED ECONOVORES

My friend Avril is a born organizer. She just has a natural knack for helping others sort and order the "stuff" in their lives. Elise Cooke, author of *Strategic Eating* (Outskirts Press, 2008), is a world-class "econovore" who achieves optimal nutrition with very little time, money or effort. Between these two experts are great ideas on how to get organized, save time and money, and stay on track nutritionally:

Buy nutrient dense foods. To get the biggest nutritional bang for your food buck, says Cooke, check the *Nutrition Facts* label. Choose products that give you the most nutrients for the price you pay, in calories as well as dollars. Nutrient-dense foods that don't break the bank include eggs, low-fat dairy foods, kale, broccoli, spinach, peanut butter, and whole wheat flour. And don't forget dried or canned beans and lentils; these are possibly the best nutritional buy in the entire supermarket.

Stock up when you find good deals on food. But only if you can safely and reasonably store what you buy, Cooke advises. "Half-price food is no savings if half of it is thrown away."

When you buy in bulk, designate separate shelves in your storage area and sort the items by category, Avril advises. Each week, transfer the foods you need to the kitchen; that way you won't forget what you have. "I have been in several homes and garages where I uncovered cases of canned, bottled and packaged food that hadn't been seen for months."

Organize food in your kitchen by category. "Then you can easily see what you have and what you need to add to your shopping list," Avril explains. Store baking items like flour, sugar and cornstarch together, for example. Organize canned goods in rows according to food groups: fruits, vegetables, beans, soups and sauces.

Moisture-proof plastic containers are a good investment for pasta, rice, and dried beans, says Avril. "They look a lot neater than those awkward bags." She also wisely suggests we place cookies and other goodies on a higher shelf, away from easy temptation.

Store coffee and tea close to your coffee maker. And keep the items you use daily, such as spices and oil, close to your cooking area. Not too close, however. Heat can destroy delicate spices and cause cooking oil to become rancid.

Sow savings. "Plant a garden and share your excess with friends... and gladly accept their extras, too," Cooke encourages. "Trade makes winners of all the participants."

Do cooperative shopping. Before you head for the store, call a friend and ask if there is anything he or she needs that you can pick up. It saves time and gasoline; and you may get a similar call someday as well.

We must also remember not to take our eyes off the nutritional ball just to save a few pennies. "You could eat dirt and save buckets of money," says Cooke. "The challenge is to eat nutritiously. Otherwise, what's the point?"

FOOD PLAN FOR EMERGENCIES

In 1989 the Loma Prieta Earthquake wiped out power to our community on the Monterey Peninsula. I was thankful at the time for the battery-powered kids' radio we had recently purchased at a garage sale for a dollar...and for the extra batteries I found stashed in a kitchen drawer.

Barbara A. Quinn, MS, RD, CDE

During those days of unexpected power outages, our young daughters thought cooking outside on the propane grill and dining by candlelight was fun. For me, it was a wake-up call to be better prepared for unexpected events.

I'm not alone. A recent Gallup poll reported that 41% of people do not have extra food and water stocked for an emergency and 27% do not have an extra supply of medicine. Both should be basic disaster preparations, says the *Federal Emergency Management Agency* (FEMA).

Here are some other ways to be ready for emergencies:

Store supplies to last two weeks. Water is the most important, say experts at FEMA. During an emergency, each person in your household will need at least one gallon of clean water every day for drinking, food preparation and hygiene. Bottled water in its original sealed container is the safest way to store this essential fluid; water stored in empty milk or juice containers can harbor bacteria.

Stock appropriate foods. We don't need more emergencies during an emergency. Stick to foods that require no refrigeration or special preparation. Check your stockpile occasionally so you can use canned goods and staples by their "Use by" dates. As you replace these items, remember "First In, First Out" which means new supplies go in the back and older items are moved forward to be used.

Store emergency foods in a dry, cool, dark area. Keep sugar, dried fruit, and nuts in screw-top jars or air-tight canisters to protect them from pests. Wrap crackers, granola bars and cookies in plastic bags and store in water-proof containers.

Use or replace foods within these general timelines:

- Six months: dry milk powder, dried fruit, crackers;
- One year: canned fruit and juice, vegetables, soup, cereal, peanut butter, jelly, hard candy, nuts, and vitamins.

- More than one year if stored properly: vegetable oils, white rice and pasta, dried beans, baking powder, salt, non-carbonated beverages, instant coffee and tea.

During an emergency, eat perishable food from the refrigerator, pantry or garden first. Tackle the freezer next. Frozen food should last at least 2 days if the door is not opened often and the interior of the food still contains ice crystals. Rely on your non-perishable foods last, after you inspect them for signs of spoilage. Toss any canned item that is swollen, dented or corroded.

Stay hydrated. We can get by on less food but not less water, say experts. During an emergency, aim to eat at least one balanced meal and drink at least 2 quarts of water each day.

FEEDING TEETH

Years ago, I remember my mom marvel at the fact that my grandmother, almost 90 years old at the time, still had all her own teeth. Times have changed...somewhat. According to the *Centers for Disease Control,* one in every four adults over the age of 65 have no natural teeth, which makes it a drag to eat corn-on-the-cob.

Why is our nutrition so important for our teeth? Because specific nutrients maintain strong teeth and strong teeth maintain our ability to get nutrients. Here's the latest on this topic from a recent position paper by the *Academy of Nutrition and Dietetics*:

Bacteria that live in our mouth love sugar. They feed on "fermentable carbohydrates" in our food and produce acids that eat away at the protective enamel on the surface of our teeth. This process weakens teeth and sets them up for decay. Yuck.

Where do fermentable carbs that pump up mouth bacteria hide out? Sugar-sweetened beverages such as soda, fruit drinks, energy drinks, and sweet tea—any food that contains added sugar—are great storehouses for these tooth-destroying carbs. Of course teeth destroying bacteria adore candies, cookies, cakes and any other sugary food. And foods that stick on the teeth longer like honey, molasses, raisins and other dried fruit are especially appetizing to mouth bacteria.

Some foods and food ingredients can *protect* our teeth from decay, however. Chew on these, say experts:

Sugar-free chewing gum. Chewing gum stimulates saliva in the mouth to bathe teeth with antibacterial agents that kill harmful acids. Mouth bacteria especially don't like to eat sugar-alcohols such as xylitol and mannitol which are often used to sweeten sugar-free gum.

Fresh fruits and vegetables. Vitamin C in these foods is crucial for the production of collagen, a protein that helps form healthy gums. And chewing on these fibrous foods stimulates the production of bacteria-fighting saliva.

Protein foods such as meat, eggs, cheese, fish, beans and legumes add strength to teeth and gums. Proteins also arm saliva with its antibacterial properties.

Whole grain, low sugar breads and cereals provide a host of nutrients that enhance our immune response to fight off pesky bacteria.

And excuse me for bringing up a controversial nutrition topic, but good evidence has shown that dental cavities can be prevented when teeth are exposed to fluoride in water, food or toothpaste. See more on this in Chapter 8.

So here's the formula to grow old with your teeth like my grandmother: Chew, chew, chew your food to stimulate saliva. Don't let sugar hang out too often with the bacteria in your mouth. And yes dear, you must brush your teeth after you eat…with a fluoride-containing toothpaste. If you can't brush right away, chew a piece of sugar-free gum. That ought'a keep those teeth in their place.

FINDING FIBER WITH TED

We were sitting on his patio one evening when I announced that I was writing a column on dietary fiber. Ted, who has developmental delays, looked at me quizzically. Do you know which foods contain fiber? I asked.

"I don't have a clue," he said flatly. "Lettuce? Celery? Tomatoes?"

Right, I said. Basically anything that begins its life in the ground has fiber..at least initially.

"I've got a question," Ted interjected. "Does milk have fiber?"

Does milk begin its life in the ground? I asked.

"Indirectly." he laughed. "Does fish have fiber?"

Remember the definition, I said. Fiber is the part of fruits, vegetables, grains and other plant-based foods that cannot be digested by our human bodies. Grains used to make bread, like wheat and rye, contain fiber. But not all bread contains fiber.

"How come they take the fiber out?" Ted asked.

Good question, why *do* they take the fiber out? It would be better for us, health-wise, if they didn't.

"How can they keep the fiber in there?" he continued.

Well, they can include all parts of the seed—the "whole grain"—when they grind it into flour for bread. That would help.

"Potatoes have fiber. Do they take it out when they make potato bread?" he asked.

Let's take a look, I said, heading for the kitchen to find the package of bread Ted had for lunch that day. We looked at the label. Let's see…dietary fiber…less than 1 gram…"

We looked at each other and in unison, said, "Booooo."

So if we want to have bread with fiber, it would be…?

"Whole grain and not refined without fiber," he answered like a real nutrition pro. "If it's too refined, they've taken the good stuff out of it. Does popcorn have fiber?"

What does it look like before you pop it?

"Kernels of corn," he said.

Bingo; popcorn is a whole grain because we eat the entire kernel after it pops. So yes, it does contain fiber.

"What's a good amount of fiber to eat?" he asked.

Most adults need at least 25 grams a day, I said. So if your bread has less than 1 gram of fiber per slice…

"You have to eat a whole loaf!"

Better yet, find a bread with more fiber per slice, I said. We did a little figuring and calculated Ted ate about 12 grams of fiber on this day. That's about half of what you need, I said. And unfortunately, that amount is about average for most Americans.

"So…I'm average," he said.

I posed one last question: Why do people need fiber?

"For their digestion? And fiber also has vitamin power, doesn't it?" Ted asked.

Some fiber helps exercise your digestive system and keeps you regular, I confirmed. Other fibers pull extra cholesterol out of your body. Vitamins are often found in foods that contain fiber, such as fruits, vegetables, beans and whole grains. And some fibers feed good bacteria in your lower intestine that help you digest vitamins and minerals. So fiber is a good thing, right?

"Right!" he said with his typical enthusiasm. "I really learned something tonight!" So did I. Thanks, Ted.

REFLECTION: Beyond their designation as "soluble" or "insoluble," dietary fibers are now categorized according to their beneficial effects. For example, "viscous" fibers like pectin found in apple peels help lower blood cholesterol and glucose levels and promote satiety. "Non-fermentable" fibers such as wheat bran keep the digestive tract moving. And "fermentable" fibers promote healthy colons by feeding the good bacteria that reside there.

NUTRITION MIXTURES

So our friend Brad, poured a wet blob of cement mixture from his truck into a frame that was soon to become a concrete slab. And I was learning how this all worked.

"Smooth it evenly back and forth," he said while he demonstrated with a tool that looked like a giant spatula.

Kind of like icing a cake? I asked.

"Kind of," he said patiently.

Cement and concrete are unique and specialized materials, I discovered from this expert. Concrete contains sand and gravel mixed with "cementing" materials such as limestone, silica and iron. Of course this got my nutrition brain thinking about these same ingredients in our human bodies. Limestone is calcium carbonate, a common ingredient in calcium supplements. Silica is a form of the trace mineral silicon, which our bodies use in tiny amounts to strengthen bones. And iron is a key ingredient in blood and muscle tissue. When consumed in the right proportions, these nutrients do indeed hold us together.

But here's an important point: Even though our bodies share some of the same cementing materials, we are not concrete slabs. And it reminded me of the flawed logic behind such statements as, "Margarine is one molecule away from being plastic."

Margarine is made from vegetable oils. Most plastics are made from crude oil that is mined from rocks; plastic can be manufactured from plant based oils as well. Trying to equate margarine with plastic is like saying plain water (H_2O) is one molecule away from hydrogen peroxide bleach (H_2O_2), according to factual review of this topic by the *Heart Foundation of New Zealand*. These two compounds share similar ingredients, but they are definitely not the same.

But I digress. We helped Brad put the finishing touches on the wet concrete and I learned that the dried slab gets stronger as it ages although it will eventually crack. The secret, he said, is to make allowances so it cracks as evenly and gracefully as possible. I'll think about that, too…

Barbara A. Quinn, MS, RD, CDE

> REFLECTION: *Soon after this column was published, I received these comments from Daniel Atkinson, Professor Emeritus of Biochemistry at the University of California, Los Angeles:*
>
> *"You call silicon a trace mineral and say silica is a 'form' of it. Actually silicon is an element rather than a mineral and is a component of the mineral silica. That isn't a particularly important error in a column such as yours.*
>
> *"But the egregious error is your characterization of silicon as a trace material. Actually silicon is the second most abundant element in the earth's crust (after oxygen), making up about one quarter of the mass of the crust. In fact it is more abundant by weight than all of the more than one hundred other elements combined (excluding oxygen, of course). Hardly a trace!"*
>
> *I do stand corrected, Dr. Atkinson. Silicon is indeed a chemical element although sometimes referred to (incorrectly, as you pointed out) as a mineral.*
>
> *While I appreciate the fact that silicon makes up a good portion of our earth's crust, it is found in only trace amounts in the human body; thus its nutritional designation as a "trace" nutrient. Nutrition researchers have established that silicon may be important to bone and heart health, but no current recommendation has yet established it as an essential nutrient.*

FARM TOUR

Woody Yerxa knows farming. Besides the ten acres of golden sunflowers he grew as a glowing backdrop for his daughter Melissa's outdoor wedding, his land produces a host of other crops as well.

For four generations, Woody's family has farmed in Colusa County, California. In addition to sunflowers, they grow walnuts, plums (the variety that is dried to make prunes), almonds, wheat, rice, alfalfa, tomatoes, cucumbers, squash, watermelon, cantaloupe, and corn.

On the morning before his daughter's wedding, Woody loaded us into his truck for a personal tour of his family's farm. As we bumped across the fields, I took note of what we learned from this seasoned farmer:

California is the nation's number one crop-producing state, Woody informed us. And 99 percent of the farms in California are family owned. "Very few actual corporations do well in farming because when you farm, you have to make quick decisions."

As we drove through field after field, I was surprised by the rich diversity of plant life. "Our land is more productive than it was 70 years ago," Woody said. "That's because we continuously work nutrients and plant matter back into the soil." Crops are carefully rotated, he explained, to keep valuable nutrients in the soil as well as control for weeds and pests.

"It costs me about $45,000 to spray one field for insects or fungus," Woody explained. "So if I don't have to spray, I don't. We rely a lot on beneficials like lady bugs that prey on crop-destroying pests."

We drove past an orchard that Woody identified as "aamon" trees. "Here in Colusa," he explained with a grin, "we harvest almonds by shaking them off trees; and that's how they get the "L" shaken out of them..."

Next on the tour were rice fields, a predominant crop in Colusa County, where I learned a new term. "Rough rice" is how rice comes from the field, wrapped in its hull. When the hull is removed, brown rice, which has an outer coating of bran, remains. Essential fats, vitamins and potent antioxidant nutrients are housed in the bran. Why then, I asked, is the bran removed from white rice?

"Because it goes rancid quickly," said Yerxa. "Rice shipped around the world often has the bran removed so it can be safely stored."

My favorite crop this day was the sprawling field of wedding sunflowers lifting their faces to the sun. Seeds harvested from these flowers are packed with fats essential for human health. And they are good sources of potent antioxidant nutrients such as vitamin E and selenium as well as zinc, iron, copper, folate and other B vitamins.

As the tour ended, Woody explained how, in many respects, farming has become high tech. His crew uses lasers to level the ground so they can use water more efficiently. And to maximize yields, they keep each row of crops razor-straight with a GPS (Global Positioning System).

Yet farmers like Yerxa still rely on nature to do much of the work. They rent bees to pollinate their crops. They recycle straw left over from the wheat harvest and sell it to mushroom farmers. And they still tend and weed many of their crops by hand. "The number one expense in farming is still labor," Woody said.

Later that day, Melissa's wedding featured many of the foods produced on her family's farm: roasted squash, onions, and mushrooms, rice salad with toasted "aamons" and crisp cucumber salad. Yum, yum, and yum; if the energy level of this family is any gauge of the healthfulness of their diet, sign me up.

REFLECTION: In 2013, I received a letter from Woody's wife, Kathy. She was delighted to report that she and Woody would soon be grandparents. She also informed me that their son Mitchell, a graduate of Cal Poly State University, has returned home to work with his dad on the family farm.

"He has been working for a year now and is doing just great," she writes. "After his first week back, he said, 'Mom, I knew in theory that we worked really hard; but until I started doing it for myself every day, I really did not understand how long the hours really are."

WHAT RANCHERS DO

What a scene. Bolts of sunshine were settling into dark clouds on the vast horizon of western Nebraska. Newborn black calves, faces splashed with white, romped and played over sprawling acres of pasture while mother cows grazed and kept watch over their babies.

I watched as my son-in-law maneuvered his giant red tractor through gate openings to deliver huge rounds of hay to his cows and their little ones. A late spring storm was brewing and Tom wanted to be sure the herd was well-supplied with food.

My job was to zoom over the bumpy landscape in a fun little all-terrain vehicle to open and close gates. But mostly I admired Tom's hard work caring for his land and cattle. When the last load of hay was delivered, I scooted over and he hopped into the driver's seat. What are we doing now? I yelled as we zipped around the pasture, right through the herd of cows and calves.

"We're looking to make sure everyone is healthy," Tom yelled back. "If babies don't jump up or run away when we get close, or aren't nursing, or have diarrhea...those are signs that they may not be well."

He should know. Besides raising beef cattle, Tom and his dad, Jim, are doctors of veterinary medicine. When it comes to animal welfare, they practice what they preach.

"Ranchers care about their animals," Tom said. "We know that stress is no better for animals than it is for humans. A happy cow is a productive cow. So we really strive to keep our animals healthy and happy. It they aren't, it comes directly out of our pocketbook."

Everyone looked happy and healthy today. Rarely do these cattle get sick. But if they do, they are separated from the herd and treated.

"Food safety is a large part of our job when it comes to food animals," Tom explained. "If I have a sick cow and I give her an antibiotic and she gets better, we know exactly how long it takes for the body to metabolize that drug and eliminate it completely from the body. So none of the meat from the animal has antibiotic residues in it. If there are, that is called adulteration and there are massive fines. It's a big deal."

"Currently, the FDA has made it so that no antibiotics can be sold for use in animals without a prescription," he continues. "And in order to get a prescription you have to have a valid relationship with a veterinarian, someone who is educated and trained in the workings of animals and food safety."

With the sun setting and the clouds darkening, Tom jumped back into his big red tractor and I whizzed ahead to open and close gates on our way back to the house. Wonder what's for dinner?

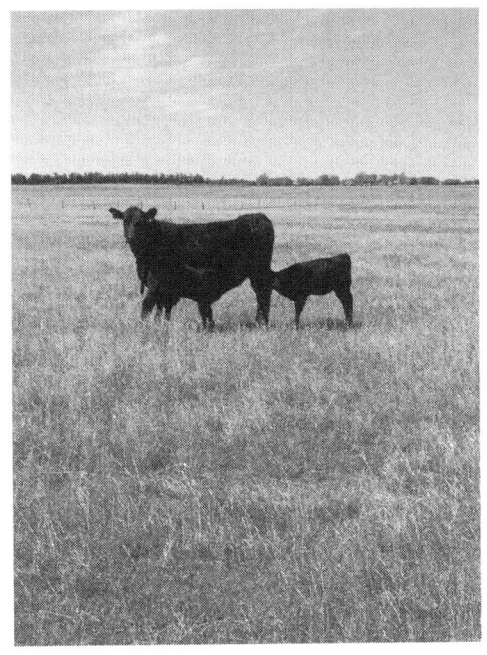

Angus cattle at the Furman Ranch, Alliance, Nebraska

OPTIMAL NUTRITION

SECRETS OF FISH

"I don't mind you writing about our trip," he said as we drove out of town. "But you can't identify the river where I'm going to fish. It's my secret spot." I nodded and jotted down a few notes. He eyed my suspiciously. "And you can't say what kind of fly I use on my fishing rod." I promised not to divulge any fly fisherman secrets.

When we arrived at (secret), we stayed with our good friends, Roy and Marge. On the first day of fishing, the guys came home with a 28-inch steelhead trout they caught at an undisclosed location.

It's no secret that fish, especially fatty fish like salmon, is a good source of omega-3 fats. Named for their chemical structure which has a double bond three carbons from the "omega" end of their carbon chain, omega-3's fats are essential for human health. "Essential" in nutrition terms means the body needs this nutrient and cannot make it internally; it must be supplied in the diet.

Why are omega-3's so necessary? Ahh, that's the secret researchers are beginning to unravel. We know omega-3 fats help form the structures of important body parts such as nerves, eyes, and brain cells. They also play a role in regulating blood pressure and cholesterol levels. Omega-3's may also help fight infections and help the body heal from injury.

A recent health claim approved by the United States Food and Drug Administration (FDA) states, "Supportive but not conclusive research shows that consumption of EPA and DHA omega-3 fatty acids may reduce the risk of coronary heart disease."

EPA and DHA are the two most active forms of omega-3 fats and the main type of fat in the thinking area of our brains, the cerebral cortex. They are primarily found in dark-fleshed fatty fish such as salmon, sardines, tuna and trout. EPA is code for ecosapentaenoic ("eco-sa-pen-ta-NO-ic") acid; DHA stands for docosahexaenoic ("doe-coe-sa-hexa-NO-ic") acid.

Another type of omega-3 fat, alpha-linolenic acid (ALA), is found primarily in plant-based foods such as flaxseed, canola oil, walnuts, wheat germ, and chia seeds.

How much omega-3 fats we need is still a bit of a mystery. It's been estimated that men need 1.6 grams and women need 1.1 grams of omega-3 fats each day. Pregnant and breastfeeding women need 1.4 and 1.3 grams daily for the development of infant eyes and brains.

Best way to get omega-3's, say health experts, is to eat fish at least two times a week. Add other sources such as ground flaxseed or walnuts to your daily diet, too. A four-ounce serving of salmon or trout provides about 1 gram (1000 milligrams) of omega-3 fatty acids, for example. If you take omega-3's in supplement form, do not exceed 2 grams (2000 milligrams) a day unless your doctor approves, says the FDA.

Of course the best part of fishin' is the eatin'. We seasoned our fresh trout with herbs and lemon and other secret ingredients and baked it in foil. Marge served it with fresh vegetables and flaxseed bread from a local bakery. No secret, it was yummy.

REFLECTION: To find the best advice on how to choose eco-friendly fish meals, check out the Monterey Bay Aquarium's Seafood Watch® website, downloadable mobile app, and pocket guide. http://www.seafoodwatch.org/cr/cr_seafoodwatch/sfw_recommendations.aspx

BENEFITS OF BERRIES

I popped another blueberry in my mouth and listened intently to the speaker. This was, after all, the "Berry Health Benefits Symposium" where researchers from around the world converged to report their findings on the health impacts of eating berries.

Scientists spoke about powerful compounds in berries such as strawberries, blueberries, raspberries, and cranberries that help protect the body from what neuroscientist Jim Joseph of Tufts University Human Research Center on Aging calls "the evil Gemini twins"---inflammation and oxidative stress. When thrown out of balance, these bodily processes damage healthy cells and lead to the development of chronic diseases like heart disease and cancer.

Heart disease and obesity, for example, are now considered "pro-inflammatory" conditions, according to Britt Burton-Freeman, PhD, obesity and metabolic disease researcher at the Illinois Institute of Technology. She reported how a high fat meal creates an inflammatory response in the body (as measured by markers in the blood called C-reactive proteins). Something as simple as adding 2/3 cup of sliced strawberries to a meal helped block this damaging inflammation. "Time and again," she said, "we continue to find substances in fruits and vegetables that work as powerful anti-inflammatory agents."

Oxidative stress is a bad boy, too. "Just look in the mirror," Dr. Joseph told us. "Wrinkles and skin damage are signs of oxidative stress." His research shows that people who eat a diet rich in fruits and vegetables are healthier as they age. "Compounds in these foods quench the fires of inflammation and prevent or reverse some age-related processes."

Will antioxidant compounds in berries make us young again? "No," said Joseph, "but they can help." One of his studies showed that the addition of blueberry juice (up to about 10 ounces a day for 12 weeks) improved memory scores in people diagnosed with mild cognitive impairment or what he jokingly referred to as "CRS" (Can't Remember Stuff).

Polyphenols for example, are the potent antioxidants found in berries (and red wine) that keep the lining inside blood vessels soft and pliable. Proanthocyanidins ("pro-antho-sigh-a-ni-dens") are antioxidants that make cells behave and can be powerful protectors against cancer, say experts.

Cranberries, for example, contain proanthocyanidins that keep bacteria from sticking to the walls of the bladder and help prevent urinary tract infections. These same substances may also help reduce the risk for stomach ulcers caused by *H. pylori* bacteria, we learned from research scientist Amy Howell of Rutgers University.

How much is needed to see health benefits? As little as one daily cup of cranberry juice, one-fourth cup of dried cranberries or a half cup of cranberry sauce can do the trick, Howell reported. And for those worried about calories and sugar, the light versions of cranberry juice were just as effective.

I piled more berries on my plate and noted these reminders:

Eat more color. Anthocyanins are the color pigments that give red, blue and purple color to strawberries, blueberries, raspberries and other berries. These compounds have been found to change biological processes within the cells that can improve memory and protect us against cancer and heart disease.

Eat the whole fruit. Berries are excellent packages of nutrients and other compounds that nourish and protect the body from everyday cellular distress, say these experts. And because they are storehouses of so many known and unknown substances that impact wellness, whole fruits are almost always superior to isolated ingredients packed into a pill.

Eat a variety. It's not just one particular compound in berries that imparts a powerful impact on health and longevity, said Ron Prior, Ph.D biochemist from Cornell University. No kidding. My head was spinning as these scientists discussed the various polyphenols, flavonoids, anthocyanins, and proanthocianidins that impart the collective health effects of berries. Fascinating, too, that each berry has a distinct profile of these antioxidant, anti-inflammatory compounds. Most researchers believe it's the synergy of these substances working together that confer the greatest benefits to our health.

Keep it in balance. Too much of even something beneficial is not good, one speaker emphasized. "Maintaining balance is a good thing," she explained as she described the "nutritional equilibrium" we achieve when we consume optimal amounts of nutrients and other protective substances in our diets.

Eat berries often. Most of the promising research shows a health effect from eating one-half to one cup of berries a day, fresh or frozen. And good news: We don't have to pronounce all the complicated substances in berries; we just need to eat them.

REFLECTION: Colorful berries continue to live up to their reputations as "super fruits." Anthocyanins are a particular type of flavonoid phytochemical responsible for the bright red-orange or blue-purple color of many fruits and vegetables. Besides their bright colors, anthocyanins have gained favor as brain boosters and intense fighters against cancer and heart disease.

ALL 'CHOKED UP

Question: What delicious food weighs three-fourths of a pound, yet has fewer calories than an apple, more potassium than a banana, and more fiber than a slice of whole grain bread?

Answer: An artichoke, which just so happens to be the official vegetable of Monterey County, California.

How do these thistles-of-the-field fit into a healthy diet? Very well, thank you. If the artichoke had a nutrition label, it would truthfully declare that this flower-vegetable is fat-free, low sodium, cholesterol-free, low calorie, and a good source of fiber and vitamin C.

One artichoke contains 25 calories, barely a blip on the daily calorie screen. Yet those few calories contain at least 15 essential nutrients, including protein, vitamins and minerals like calcium and iron.

For those in the pregnant or planning-to-be-pregnant category, take note that artichokes are a tasty source of folate (folic acid). This B-vitamin is essential for babies-in-development and can help prevent a category of birth disorders known as neural tube defects.

How do you cook these funny-looking vegetables? No worries. If you can boil water, you can cook artichokes. In my book, that ranks them right up there with potatoes and other foods that don't stress my culinary skills. Here is some guidance from the *California Artichoke Advisory Board:*

Prepare: Wash artichoke under cool running water. Pull off lower petals and cut off stem. If desired, trim tips of petals. Plunge artichoke into water acidified with lemon, white wine, or club soda to preserve the green color.

Boil. Place prepared artichokes in pan just large enough to hold them upright. Add water to cover. Add one ounce (about two tablespoons) lemon juice per quart of water and a small amount of oil if preferred. Cover and bring to a boil. Reduce heat and simmer 25 to 40 minutes, depending on size of artichoke, or until petal near the center pulls out easily. Pour off water and stand artichoke upside down to drain.

Steam. Place prepared artichokes on rack over an inch or two of boiling water. Cover and cook 25 to 40 minutes or until petals near center pull out easily.

Quinn-Essential Nutrition

Microwave. To prepare an artichoke for an individual serving, invert prepared artichoke in deep one-quart microwave-safe container. Add 3 tablespoons of water, 1 teaspoon lemon juice, and a teaspoon of vegetable oil if desired. Cover with heavy-duty plastic wrap and prick with a fork to allow steam to escape. Cook on high power 6 to 8 minutes or until petal near center pulls out easily. Allow to stand for 5 minutes.

Perhaps the only thing not to like about artichokes is the cost. Large 'chokes may sell for as much as a dollar each. But look what you get for your buck; food you can eat with your fingers, a conversation piece for guests who have never seen such a thing, and some of the longest-lasting 25 calories you will ever enjoy.

PREBIOTICS AND PROBIOTICS

Once upon a time there was a great body. Inside this body lived teeny tiny "micro" organisms. Some of these organisms were friendly and some were not so friendly. But as long as the nice microbes outnumbered the not nice ones, life in the body was good. These good bacteria protected the body from intestinal infections and helped it stay in a state referred to as "regular." This encouraged the body to consume more foods that contained these beneficial organisms. Identified on food labels as "live and active cultures," these friendly bacteria became known as "probiotics."

One day it occurred to the body that these bacteria—like all living things—need to be fed. "What shall I feed my probiotic buddies so they will be fruitful and continue to multiply?" he said.

A bit of research revealed that probiotics thrive on various types of undigested fiber material from plant foods such as bananas, onions, wheat, artichokes and garlic. These so-called "fermentable fibers" are the perfect food for probiotics. and are therefore named "prebiotics."

The body found many types of prebiotics to feed the friendly microorganisms in his gut. Some were named for their chemical structure, such as oligosaccharides (oh-lee-go-sack-a-rides) and fructooligosaccharides (fruc-toe-oh-lee-go-sack-a-rides) or FOS.

Other fermentable fibers, such as inulin and resistant starches, also nourished his good gut bacteria. Soon the body noticed that these ingredients were sometimes added to certain foods and supplements. For example, some brands of milk and yogurt contain short-chain FOS and short- or long-chain inulin,. These types of prebiotics can aid digestion and the absorption of nutrients such as calcium. Some cereal and snack bars contain added inulin and oligofructose prebiotic fibers. Short chain FOS and inulin are also found in various supplements such as *Nutraflora FOS* and *FiberChoice.*

Some products contain both prebiotics *and* probiotics. Yogurt with added FOS is one example. These are referred to as "symbiotics" to designate that the two work together for good.

As the body began to feel more regular, he sought the proper dosage of prebiotics to feed the probiotics residing in his gut. According to an article on this topic in the *Academy of Nutrition and Dietetics,* the minimum dose for a prebiotic effect is 500 milligrams (one half of a gram). And the dosage for most health benefits ranges from 3 grams per day for short-chain fructooligosaccharides (FOS) to 8 grams for short- and long-chain inulin.

The body was suddenly aware there is a lot to understand about prebiotics and probiotics. One new resource on this topic is *Gut Insight,* a book and website by registered dietitian Jo Ann Hattner. www.gutinsight.com. And life was very, very good.

REFLECTION: Nutrition science continues to explore the depths of our gut flora through the Human Microbiome Project. It's a whole new area of nutrition research that is seeking to understand how specific gut flora, beneficial microorganisms that live in our intestinal tract, affect our health.

There's plenty to understand. According to a recent article in the Journal of the Academy of Nutrition and Dietetics, people with normal digestion tend to have different types of gut bacteria than people with irritable bowel syndrome (IBS) and other digestive disorders. Even our ability to gain or lose weight may be influenced by the type and amount of bacteria in our intestines, according to preliminary research. Wow.

So what do bacteria in our intestines have to do with nutrition? Plenty. The foods we eat affect the flora that grows in our gut. And the flora that grows in our gut can impact our health, say researchers.

Here's one explanation for how it works: Dietary fiber travels through the body pretty much undisturbed. When it reaches the lower end of the digestive tract (the colon), it becomes food for the friendly microbes (probiotics) that live there. These bacteria ferment the fiber and produce short chain fatty acids, substances that nourish and preserve cells in the colon and the liver. It's this process, say researchers, that may protect the body from gastrointestinal diseases as well as cancer and heart disease.

All gut bacteria is not created equal, however. My microbiota is different from your microbiota, say experts. And our gut bacteria is altered by the types of foods we eat.

For example, people who eat a high fiber diet, rich in vegetables, fruit, whole grains, beans, and nuts, tend to have a more diverse variety of gut microflora, according to nutrition professor Megan Baumler, PhD, RD. (Good bacteria in our colon, remember, thrive on dietary fiber.) And a thriving assortment of these microorganisms in the gut is considered very beneficial.

We can also eat foods or take supplements that contain "probiotics" (beneficial bacteria) or "prebiotics" (plant fibers that feed gut flora), says researcher Peter Beyer, MS, RD. Cultured dairy foods like yogurt or kefir contain probiotics for example. And we are beginning to learn how various probiotics are specific to certain health conditions. Fascinating.

Stress can disrupt the level of healthy gut bacteria in our gut, say experts. All the better to continue eating a high fiber plant-based diet during times of stress, they advise.

Research from the lab of Dr. Jeffrey Gordon from Washington University School of Medicine in St. Louis found that lean and obese people actually harbor different gut microbes that may impact weight. The benefits of these bacterial colonies appear to be linked to the quality of the diet, however; high in fruits and vegetables and low in saturated fat appears to be most beneficial.

G IS FOR GARLIC

G is for Garlic, the pungent plant with health benefits we are just beginning to understand. **G** may also remind us that Gilroy (California) is considered the "Garlic Capital of the World" and home to the annual Gilroy Garlic Festival.

A stands for allicin ("ah-LIS-in,"), the active ingredient responsible for garlic's health benefits. Allicin also gives garlic its potent aroma—what your nose picks up when you drive through Gilroy. Allicin has also been found to work like an antibiotic to fight infections.

Ever notice that you don't smell fresh garlic until it's crushed? That's because garlic has a Superman-like complex. Freshly picked, it is mild mannered with few special powers. Under pressure however, when garlic is chopped, smashed or chewed, it releases a super scent and life-sustaining actions. We may never apologize for garlic breath again; it is proof that allicin is active and at work for our benefit.

Garlic also contains a compound with blood-thinning properties called "ajoene" ("UH-ho-ene"). High doses of garlic can therefore increase the effects of anti-coagulant medications such as warfarin (*Coumadin*) or aspirin.

R is for raw...or really fresh. Only in this form does garlic have its proven health benefits. Allicin (the Superman ingredient) is so unstable that it may be non-existent in even the most carefully dried products, according to research by the late Varro E. Tyler, PhD pharmacologist at Purdue University. One exception may be dried garlic tablets or capsules which have been enteric-coated to protect garlic's active ingredients from the action of stomach acids.

Wouldn't it be easier to just chew on fresh garlic? Yes, it would; and it would be effective, too. Chewing releases the active ingredients directly into the mouth, a surefire method to receive the beneficial effects of this potent plant bulb.

L is for lower cholesterol, one of the proven benefits of eating garlic. One study suggests you need to eat 5 to 20 cloves a day to get this effect. Other experts say one fresh clove of garlic a day may still confer some benefit on cholesterol levels. Eat as much garlic as you find palatable, say most experts.

I stands for intrigued investigators, researchers impressed with garlic as a health food. Along with five other plants (flax, licorice, soybeans, citrus fruits, and root vegetables), garlic is one of the first foods to be studied by the *National Cancer Institute* for its role in cancer prevention. And it's not the vitamins or minerals in these foods that perk the interest of scientists. It is the class of substances called "phytochemicals," biological compounds found in plants, that have been found to possess important medicinal properties.

C is for caution with certain garlic preparations. Garlic packed in oil has little, if any, health benefit. That's because its active ingredient, allicin, is not stable in oil. Oil-packed garlic with no preservatives may also harbor deadly botulism spores. Be extremely cautious if you come across garlic-in-oil preparations that do not contain preservatives such as citric or phosphoric acid.

Barbara A. Quinn, MS, RD, CDE

FAQ'S ABOUT CHILE

"What are you going to do with all these chiles?" my friend Amanda asked as I loaded a giant box of fresh Hatch green chiles in her car.

I'm going to roast them...and put them in my freezer, I said.

"All of them?" she said with disbelief.

It's only 30 pounds. When I lived in New Mexico, we roasted a 50-pound sack every year.

I didn't expect her to understand. She's from California. And although this 6th Annual Green Chile Roast was held in Los Gatos (California), most of us in attendance were alumni of New Mexico State University (NMSU).

It was a nostalgic afternoon. Decades had passed since I last spoke to Dr. Garrey Carruthers, former governor of New Mexico and currently the President of NMSU. I knew Dr. Carruthers during my college years when he served as the faculty advisor to our intercollegiate rodeo team. Later when he became governor of New Mexico, I visited him in Santa Fe to encourage his signature on a licensing bill for registered dietitians.

"Did I veto it?" he joked when I reminded him of our last meeting.

You signed it, I said.

Later in the day, when Dr. Carruthers was formally introduced to our California-based alumni group, he reminded us that California was once part of New Mexico territory. "Greetings from the homeland," he announced.

He also informed us that NMSU is home to the *Chile Pepper Institute,* an international organization devoted to education and research related to chile peppers. When I got home—and after I roasted my green chile—I found these answers to common questions about our beloved chile:

Is it called "chile" or "chili?" According to the *Chile Pepper Institute,* the word "chile" comes from the Aztec "chilli" that was later changed to "chile" by Spanish-speaking Mexicans and to "chili" in some parts of the United States. In New Mexico, "chile"

Quinn-Essential Nutrition

describes the plant, as in, "Do you want red or green chile on your enchilada?" "Chili" describes what they might eat in Texas—a dish made with meat, beans, tomatoes and chile powder.

What makes chile hot? Capsaicin ("cap-SAY-sin") is the fiery component in chile peppers. This natural irritant can cause a burning sensation on any part of the body it touches. Many humans, including most who reside in New Mexico, consider this a pleasant feeling.

In what part of the chile plant is capsaicin most potent? Not in the seeds, as you might assume. Most of the capsaicin hot stuff is in the white pith of the inner wall of the chile, where the seeds are attached.

What is the hottest chile in the world? As of 2012, it's the "Trinidad Moruge Scorpion" (ouch), according to research conducted at NMSU. How hot *is* it? This chile contains enough capsaicin to burn through latex gloves, say brave researchers.

Any nutritional value to chile peppers? You bet. Chile is rich in vitamin C and beta carotene, potent antioxidants which help protect the cells of our body from damage. By the way, green chile and red chile are the same plant. Green chiles turn red as they ripen. And red chiles contain more vitamin C than the less ripe green chiles.

What will I do with 30 pounds of roasted green chiles? Chop them up to make salsa. Add them to my green chile stew. Spice up scrambled eggs...and everything else that needs a kick of flavor and nutrition.

Anything else? Why yes: A 2006 article in *Nature* magazine reported that the venom of a certain species of tarantula (a poisonous spider) activates the same pain pathway that is activated by capsaicin. Just sayin"...

Why do New Mexicans make such a big deal about their green and red chile? I guess you just have to live there.

> REFLECTION: Dr. David J. Braden, a 5*th* generation Texan, wrote in response to this column, "Hey ho, I enjoyed your recent article on my favorite vegetable. However, your mistaken reference that 'chili' is what they might eat in Texas—a dish made with meat, beans, tomatoes and chile powder,' is totally wrong. In Texas, it's not just meat; turkey or chicken won't do. Texans NEVER use beans or tomatoes. Seasonings vary, but are kept simple. And we never but never use so-called "chile powder."
> Respectfully noted.

HERBS AND SPICES

What is the difference between an herb and a spice? According to the *International Food Information Council* (IFIC), an herb is the leaf of a plant that is used for its "aromatic" properties. Spices are seasonings from other parts of the plant, such as cinnamon bark, clove buds, cumin seeds and ginger root. Besides giving flavor to food, seasonings have historically been used to preserve food, says the IFIC. And now we know they help preserve our health as well.

Cinnamon may help control diabetes. Some studies have shown that cinnamon may help lower blood glucose levels and may improve blood cholesterol levels. Other studies are not so sure. At any rate, cinnamon tastes good, is safe to use and provides great flavor to food without adding calories or carbohydrates that can raise blood sugar levels. (I like to sprinkle it over ground coffee before brewing.)

Ginger may help settle a sick tummy. My mom wisely offered me ginger ale when I had a stomach ache. And the IFIC reports that ginger has been shown to be helpful in the treatment of nausea, especially during pregnancy. Ginger may also be useful in the treatment of inflammatory conditions such as rheumatoid arthritis.

And the active ingredient in ginger called "gingerol" has shown promise in animal studies to protect against certain types of cancer.

Curry is a health food. Tumeric is a spice found in curry powder which gets its yellow color from a pigment called "curcumin." Curcumin is a potent antioxidant and is being studied for its potential protective role against Alzheimer's disease. Tumeric, which contains curcumin, is useful as a spice as well as a preservative and coloring agent in foods, says the IFIC.

Hot peppers do more than just make us sweat. When we perspire after eating hot chile peppers, we are also burning calories and fat, says the IFIC. That's due to capsaicin, the active ingredient that makes hot foods hot. In addition to making us sizzle, some studies suggest that capsaicin contributes to satiety, that feeling of satisfaction we get after a good meal. And that may keep us from overeating. Pass the chile, please.

Some seasonings protect food from bad bugs. Common spices known for their antibacterial properties include garlic, clove, cinnamon, thyme, oregano and rosemary.

There's only one drawback. These mini-vegetables-in-a-jar only perk up our lives if we take them *off* the shelf and *add* them to our food.

REFLECTION: We know that excess salt (sodium) can squeeze up blood pressure, disable kidney function, and weaken bones. Yet it's a challenge to make food taste good without it. Here's what culinary experts recommend: Combine acids such as lemon, lime or vinegar with spices to add flavor to dishes without the salt. For example, mix basil, oregano, parsley, and garlic with red wine vinegar to spice up Italian food. Deliziosa!

Food experts also say spices with similar colors seem to compliment each other taste-wise. Cinnamon and nutmeg, for instance; or garlic with lemon.

Barbara A. Quinn, MS, RD, CDE

SPICE UP YOUR LIFE

There really is a health benefit when we add spices to our food, say nutrition researchers. Besides adding good taste to meals that are good for us, herbal seasonings are surprising sources of antioxidants, natural plant substances that protect cells in our bodies from the damage that comes from every day living.

It's been estimated that we can double or triple the health value of a meal just by seasoning our food liberally with herbs and spices. (Salt and sodium-free, please.) These tiny bursts of flavor contain virtually no calories and can be powerful allies against life's daily stresses.

Seasonings can't help us when they sit in our cabinets for years and years, however. According to experts, most dried herbs and spices will retain their potency for one to three years if they are stored in airtight containers away from heat, moisture and direct sunlight. By the way, if your spice rack holds any seasoning in its original tin container (except black pepper), it's probably at least 20 years old, say experts.

When it comes to remembering what seasonings go with what foods, I'm not the spiciest herb in the cabinet. So here are some simple suggestions from the McCormick folks to deliver a healthful Mediterranean flair to our food:

- Stir ½ teaspoon oregano leaves and 1 to 2 tablespoons reduced fat feta cheese into ½ cup bottled vinaigrette salad dressing. Viola! Greek vinaigrette.
- Sauté 1 pound of sliced mushrooms in 1 tablespoon olive oil. Sprinkle with 1 teaspoon thyme leaves. (Thyme brings out the flavor of mushrooms.)
- Add rosemary leaves to vegetables like asparagus, spinach, and tomatoes.
- Mix up a batch of Mediterranean spiced olive oil: 1/4 cup olive oil, 1 teaspoon grated Parmesan cheese, ½ teaspoon garlic powder, 1/8 teaspoon crushed red pepper and a dash of sea salt. Pour into a small shallow dish and serve with bread. Yum!

Other tips from McCormick: Use whole spices in longer cooking recipes like soups and stews because they take longer to release their flavors. Use ground spices in recipes with shorter cooking times or add them near the end of cooking.

Fresh or dried? Some antioxidant compounds (such as vitamin C) are higher in fresh herbs. Others, known as "phenolic compounds" may be higher in dried herbs because they are more concentrated. Use both!

REFLECTION: In 2012, the USDA Nutrient Data Laboratory (NDL) withdrew its use of the well-known ORAC (oxygen radical absorbance capacity) scale that measured the antioxidant capacity of fruits and vegetables. Mounting evidence showed that ORAC values derived in the laboratory did not reflect the actual effects of these compounds in human health.

No worries. There is still plenty of evidence to support the addition of seasonings to our food. A 2010 study in the American Journal of Clinical Nutrition reported that a spice blend of rosemary, oregano, ginger, paprika, garlic, cloves, pepper and cinnamon added to hamburger meat before cooking reduced the concentration of malondialdehyde, a product of fat oxidation that may play a role in heart disease and cancer.

Rosemary has been found to have strong antioxidant capabilities which benefit the function of the heart as well as the brain, say scientists. Garlic, too, possesses antioxidant properties that benefit heart health. Garlic's active ingredient, allicin, is most potent when we consume fresh garlic within 10 to 45 minutes after it is cut or crushed.

A study at the University of Georgia in 2010 found that 1/4 to 1/2 teaspoon of ginger—raw or heat-treated—helped ease muscle and joint pain after strenuous exercise. Some nutrition experts recommend adding ginger to green tea or lemonade for full flavor as well as health benefits.

Cinnamon continues to be studied for its effects on blood sugars. A small study in the November 2012 Journal of the

Barbara A. Quinn, MS, RD, CDE

> *Academy of Nutrition and Dietetics reported that 6 grams (about 1 teaspoon) of ground cinnamon added to a meal of hot cereal significantly reduced the expected rise in blood sugar after that meal. Although these people did not have diabetes, the results were promising for normal- and overweight subjects.*
>
> *Keep in mind that one teaspoon of dried seasoning is equivalent in potency to two to three teaspoons of fresh herbs or spices. Both forms however, have been found to retain their antioxidant properties.*

A DOZEN FACTS ABOUT NUTS

Yes, there are a lot of nuts out there. And they can impact our health. This quiz is adapted from a "nutty test" that appeared in a recent *Wellness Letter* from the University of California at Berkeley. Additional information comes from the *International Tree Nut Council* which encourages us to "Go nuts every day!"

1. To get the health benefits of nuts, you need to: a) own a walnut orchard; b) eat about an ounce of nuts a day; c) not eat the whole can of honey-roasted peanuts. Answer: b.
2. One ounce is the same as a) 14 walnut halves; b) 19 pecan halves; c) 24 almonds; d) 49 pistachios. Answer: All are correct.
3. In more than 30 randomized controlled trials, nuts have been shown to: a) lower total cholesterol; b) lower LDL cholesterol; c) lower hunger. All are correct and attributed to the protein, fiber, and healthful fats contained in nuts.
4. Regular nut eaters tend to be a) thinner; b) less likely to have diabetes; c) more fun at parties. Answer: a, b.
5. True or False. Nut butters have the same nutritional advantages as whole nuts. Answer: True...*if* the nut butters are just ground up nuts. Check the label for unneeded sugar, salt, or unhealthy trans fat.

Quinn-Essential Nutrition

6. A whole day's supply of selenium, a potent antioxidant mineral, can be found in a) western Nebraska; b) one Brazil nut; c) 55 micrograms. Answers: b, c. (Caution: selenium can be toxic in doses higher than 400 micrograms a day.)
7. Macadamia nuts are named for a) the macadamia bird that eats them; b) John McAdam, the man who first cultivated these nuts; c) the Hawaiian word for "yummy when covered with chocolate." Answer: b.
8. Compared to other nuts, almonds contain more a) calcium; b) fiber; c) advertising from the Almond Board. Answer: All are correct.
9. English walnuts a) were never grown commercially in England; b) were first cultivated in California by Franciscan fathers; c) contain the highest amount of healthful omega-3 fats of any nut. Answer: All are correct.
10. The "Pistachio Principle" is: a) a school administrator who likes to eat nuts; b) a method demonstrated by Dr. James Painter, a behavioral eating expert from Eastern Illinois University, that fools us to eat less and feel full faster; c) the act of taking nuts (such as pistachios) out of their shells and eating them one by one. Answers: b,c.
11. Peanuts are a) legumes that think they are nuts; b) a better choice at the ball park than hotdogs; c) a good source of resveratrol, the health-promoting compound found also in red wine. Answer: all are correct.
12. Nutritionally, the best nuts are: a) unsalted; b) a variety of all kinds; c) eaten one ounce at a time. Answer: all are correct.

REFLECTION: Enjoy your nuts. Among other benefits, they are rich in an amino acid called arginine from which the body makes nitric oxide, a substance that maintains the health and flexibility of our arteries.

Barbara A. Quinn, MS, RD, CDE

SOYBEANS AND THE SCIENCE OF PLUTO

It was the only astronomy course I took at New Mexico State University. And it was memorable. Our professor was noted astronomer, Dr. Clyde Tombaugh, best known for his discovery of Pluto. Our esteemed professor required his students to spend one evening each week staring up at the heavens from behind the chemistry building, where the lights of campus were dimmed enough for us to see the constellations.

I especially remember the last week of class when Dr. Tombaugh described his painstaking process to identify Pluto, visible as one tiny dot among millions of other tiny dots spread across the vast solar system.

In 2006, years after Dr. Tombaugh's amazing discovery, Pluto was downgraded from its planet status to "dwarf planet." That's science for you; we change our thinking as we gather new facts. In 1999 for example, research suggested that increased intake of soy protein lowered "bad" LDL cholesterol levels in the blood. This was enough evidence to convince the United States Food and Drug Administration (FDA) to approve a health claim that stated, "25 grams of soy protein a day, as part of a diet low in saturated fat and cholesterol, may reduce the risk for heart disease."

More recently however, a review of more than 20 clinical trials concluded that the benefits of soy may not be as profound as we once thought. According to the Science Advisory Committee of the American Heart Association, soy protein may lower cholesterol levels about 3 percent—less than previously estimated. This committee also found that supplements of isoflavones, active ingredients in soybeans, did not have significant benefits for heart health.

Soy has also fallen from favor in the hot flash department. Recent clinical trials found no significant improvements in menopause symptoms when women took supplements of soy isoflavones. And the latest research findings on the effect of soy in slowing bone loss have been mixed, meaning some studies found a benefit and others did not.

Pluto still stays in orbit although our understanding of this celestial body planet has changed. So too, the basic facts about soy foods have not changed. Considered the highest quality protein of any plant food, soybeans are rich in fiber, vitamins and minerals and still considered an important health food.

REFLECTION: In 2013, research confirmed the safety and protective effects of soy foods in relation to cancer risk. Human studies—as opposed to earlier studies on rodents—have shown that soy foods are safe, even for women with a history of breast cancer.

Some studies, says Marji McCullough, ScD, RD of the American Cancer Society, have shown that regular soy consumption may decrease a woman's risk for cancer recurrence. Whole soy foods (such as soybeans, tofu, edamame, or soy milk) are recommended over soy supplements, however. Also remember that fermented soy foods such as miso or soy sauce are high in sodium.

Nutrition scientists aren't the only ones to change their views because of new evidence. In September 2014, the Harvard-Smithsonian Center for Astrophysics voted that Pluto is indeed a planet in its own right.

REDUCING THE RISKS

NUTRIENTS TO BOOST IMMUNITY

"A vitamin is a substance that makes you ill if you don't eat it," said Albert Szent-Gyorgyi, winner of the Nobel Prize in Physiology or Medicine in 1937. He understood what we now know: Deficiencies of vitamins and other vital nutrients can cause us to fall prey to illness.

So do our food choices really influence how susceptible we are to sickness? You bet your sweet pepper they do. Specific nutrients in foods can indeed enhance our immunity, the ability of our bodies to stay well. Here are some with special powers, according to the *Academy of Nutrition and Dietetics* and other nutrition experts:

Protein: Our immune cells that fight off infections and other unwelcome invaders are made of protein. High quality sources include fish, poultry, lean beef and pork, fish, eggs, beans and soy foods.

Vitamin A: Ever wonder why moms of old dosed their darlings with cod liver oil? Among other components, this fish oil is a good source of vitamin A, an essential nutrient that helps maintain the mucosal cells that line our intestines and lungs. These organs act as sentries to guard us from disease-causing invaders. Carrots, kale, spinach, sweet potatoes and red bell peppers are good sources of vitamin A..or beta-carotene, which safely converts to vitamin A in the body.

Vitamin C: Although scientists still don't understand the exact way that vitamin C works to boost immune function, we do know this essential vitamin plays an important role in healing wounds and strengthening our resistance to disease. Vitamin C also helps form antibodies that fight off infection. Since this essential nutrient is easily destroyed by air, heat and prolonged storage, aim to eat at least one high vitamin C food each day. Sources include oranges, grapefruit, strawberries, tomatoes, peppers, kiwifruit, broccoli and Brussels sprouts.

Zinc: Like an army that relies on a continual renewal of supplies and soldiers, our immune system relies on zinc to consistently renew disease-fighting cells. And since zinc is bound to protein in food, it makes sense that zinc is found in protein-containing foods such as oysters, beef, pork, liver, whole grains, beans, nuts and seeds. Interestingly, zinc has been called "the essential toxin" due to the fact that is it is required for optimal health yet can actually impair immune function when consumed in excess.

Vitamin E: Given its antioxidant ability to neutralize free radicals, vitamin E keeps the machinery of the immune system functioning at capacity. Good sources include nuts, seeds, and whole grains; wheat germ is an especially good source.

Are multivitamin/mineral supplements a good idea? They are if we consistently miss out on major nutrient groups in our usual diets. Whether or not to take a daily vitamin and mineral supplement is a discussion worth having with your health provider.

WHEN GOOD FOOD GOES BAD

It was nasty; a piece of chicken had been forgotten in the back of the refrigerator since the Stone Age. And because it was entombed in a plastic container, my usually sensitive sniffer did not tip me off. Noses are not the best way to determine if a food is safe to eat anyway; bad bugs can attack our food unnoticed.

Even organically grown food is susceptible to bacteria, molds, viruses and parasites when conditions are right. Teeny tiny microorganisms can enter the body anywhere along the food chain, from the field to the store to our kitchen.

How can we keep our food safe to eat? Here are some recommendations from the US Center for Food Safety and Applied Nutrition (CFSAN) and the Centers for Disease Control (CDC):

- Be choosy. Select fruits and vegetables that are not damaged or bruised. Bacteria hide in bruised and battered spots.
- Stay cool. Do not buy produce that is already cut (such as melon) unless it is refrigerated or displayed on ice.
- Wash your hands in warm soapy water before handling food.
- Wash all produce under clean running water before eating, even those with skins you peel such as oranges and melons. Most experts advise against using soap and detergents to wash produce. Gently scrub foods with edible skins such as potatoes or summer squash. For vegetables such as lettuce and cabbage, remove the outer leaves before you wash them. And wait to wash your produce until right before you prepare them to eat; this preserves them longer.
- Label a DCB (Designated Cutting Board) to be used only for fresh fruits and vegetables. Always use a separate cutting board for raw meats, poultry and seafood. Wash all cutting boards, utensils and countertops with hot soapy water; then sanitize with a solution of 1 teaspoon chlorine bleach in 1 quart of water.
- Transport vegetable or fruit salads in ice-packed containers. Refrigerate any leftovers within two hours; otherwise, toss them.

And don't forget to check the back of your refrigerator from time to time.

Quinn-Essential Nutrition

REFLECTION: *Ever wonder what those dates on perishable foods such as meat, poultry, eggs, and dairy products mean? Here are the official definitions:*

"Sell-By" *tells the store how long to display the product for sale; we can safely buy the food by that date.*

"Best If Used By (or Before)" *is the date by which we should consume the food for best flavor and quality. It may not be a hazard by that date, however.*

"Use-By" *is the latest date to use the product for peak quality as per the manufacturer.*

WARD OFF MEMORY LOSS

"Something's not right with my brain," my dad told me the year before he was diagnosed with Alzheimer's disease, the most common cause of dementia that destroys the ability of nerves to carry messages to the brain. Dad was in his 70's at the time and up to this point had always possessed a sharp memory.

We may sometimes forget things as we get older, but dementia is not a part of normal aging, say experts from Alzheimer's Disease International (ADI) which released the World Alzheimer Report in 2014. Numerous research studies now demonstrate that we can reduce our risk for developing dementia if we choose healthier lifestyles, say the experts who compiled this data. Here are some of their key recommendations:

Take care of your heart. What's good for our heart is also very good for our brain. Strategies that control blood cholesterol and other markers of heart disease benefit our brains as well.

Don't smoke. After the age of 65, ex-smokers have the same risk of dementia as people who have never smoked. Those who continue to smoke, however, have a much higher risk for brain malfunctions.

Keep your blood pressure under control. Raised blood pressure in our middle years of life is associated with a "considerable increase in risk for dementia in late life," stated one reviewer of this report.

Be physically active. Energetic bodies keep brains lively as well, say researchers. Although we need more study in this area, exercise appears to improve the function of nerves and memory transmitters in the brain.

Eat a healthy diet. Most promising to ward off dementia appears to be the Mediterranean-type of diet, say researchers. This eating style—rich in cereals, fruits, fish, legumes, and vegetables—supplies key nutrients that nourish the brain. Omega-3 fats from fish and B-vitamins from grains and legumes help support and maintain brain function. Fruits and vegetables supply a host of antioxidant nutrients that protect message-carrying neurons in the brain.

Keep your blood glucose (sugar) levels under control. People with diabetes have a 50% increased chance to develop dementia later in life, according to this report.

Challenge your brain. Mentally stimulating activities throughout life can help ward off the development of dementia later in life.

Enjoy social activities. I like this recommendation; it's based on evidence that shows we can lessen our risk for dementia when we take pleasure in life with others.

Keep learning. Education in early life and beyond is strongly protective against dementia.

This report also reminds me that aging is gift. I'll try to remember that.

Quinn-Essential Nutrition

CHOLESTEROL QUIZ

This quiz reminds us that September is a) Healthy Aging Month; b) National Cholesterol Education Month; b) National Breakfast Month; d) Fruit and Veggies—More Matters Month. Answer: All are correct...really.

Fall is a good time to a) think about the holidays; b) get your cholesterol numbers checked; c) eat a healthy breakfast; d) eat more apples, tomatoes, and zucchini. Answer: Yes.

According to statistics from the Centers for Disease Control and Prevention (CDC), one of the main risk factors for heart disease and stroke is a) the presidential election; b) zucchini bread; c): abnormal levels of cholesterol in the blood. Answer: c.

High blood cholesterol can a) be a walking time-bomb; b) cause "hardening of the arteries"; c) block the flow of blood to the heart. All are correct.

The two main causes for high blood cholesterol levels are a) Thanksgiving and Christmas; b) genetics and lifestyle; c) Democrats and Republicans. Answer: b.

Saturated fat a) saturates your body with fat; b) can cause a rise in "bad" LDL cholesterol; c) is easy to identify on a food label. Answer: b, c

People with diabetes or heart disease are wise to a) eat more vegetables; b) eat no more than 2 egg yolks a week; c) not order buttered popcorn at the movies. All are correct.

Strategies that can reduce high cholesterol levels include: a) sew your mouth shut; b) eat more soluble fiber; c) exercise for at least 30 minutes on most days. Answer: b, c.

Soluble fiber is a substance in a) giant Slurpees; b) cooked beans; c) oats; d) apples. Answer: b, c, d.

In medical circles, "TLC" stands for a) Take Less Cream; b) Treat LDL Cholesterol; c) Therapeutic Lifestyle Changes to reduce the risk for heart disease. Answer c.

Proven lifestyle changes that can reduce dangerous levels of blood cholesterol include: a) lose weight; b) lose the remote control; c) eat 4 to 5 cups of fruits and vegetables every day. Answer: All are correct.

"BOLD" stands for a) Beware Of Little Donuts; b) Beef in an Optimal Lean Diet; b) a recent clinical trial that showed lean beef can be safely included in diets that lower cholesterol. Answer: b, c.

Omega-3 fats in fish have been studied for their ability to a) leap giant buildings in a single bound; b) lower "bad" LDL cholesterol and triglycerides; c) prevent heart attacks. Answer: b, c.

The American Heart Association recommends we eat more a) fruits and vegetables; b) poultry, fish and nuts; c) low fat dairy products. All are correct.

Nuts and avocados are a) high in healthy monounsaturated fat; b) good replacements for foods high in saturated fat; c) yummy in salads. All are correct.

REFLECTION: Debate between high fat and low fat proponents continues. A systematic review and meta-analysis of 32 randomized controlled trials in the December 2013 issue of the Journal of the Academy of Nutrition and Dietetics reported that lower fat diets produced more pronounced falls in total and "bad" LDL cholesterol levels. On the other hand, high fat diets resulted in more distinct rises in total cholesterol and "good" HDL cholesterol as well as decreases in blood triglyceride levels.

Lower cholesterol levels were also associated with diets that were lower in saturated fat (primarily from high fat meat and dairy foods) and higher in polyunsaturated fat from plant-based oils and fish. Beneficial HDL cholesterol levels were seen more with higher intakes of monounsaturated fats such as olive and canola oils, avocados, nuts and nut oils. In addition, unhealthful rises in blood triglyceride levels were associated with higher intakes of carbohydrates, sugars and starches.

ANSWERS ABOUT SALT

Salt preserves and enhances the flavor of food. It suppresses bitterness. We hold in high regard those who are "the salt of the earth" and "worth their salt." Sodium, which makes up half of the salt molecule known a sodium chloride, is important for our health. Our bodies need sodium to balance fluid levels. It is also required to transmit nerve impulses and for the normal function of active muscles.

Somewhere along the way, however, we got too much of a good thing. Excessive intake of sodium contributes to adverse blood pressure, the abnormal force of blood against the walls of the arteries that can lead to stroke, heart failure or kidney disease. Take this quiz to see how much you really know about salt and sodium:

1. Salt is a) half sodium and half chloride; b) good on popcorn; c) a bigger contributor to high blood pressure than sodium or chloride alone. Answers: All are correct.
2. In salt history, the *Morton* "Umbrella Girl" promoted the phrase: a) "When it rains, it pours;" b) "A little dab'll do ya;" c) "Please pass the biscuits." Answer a.

3. According to the US Centers for Disease Control, 9 out of 10 Americans a) have spices in their cabinets more than six years old; b) eat too much sodium; c) aren't worth their weight in salt. Answer: b.
4. Excessive salt in the diet can interfere with a) the effectiveness of blood pressure medications; b) meaningful relationships; c) kidney function. Answers: a, c.
5. The fact that canned spinach contains over twice the sodium of fresh spinach shows that a) Popeye probably had high blood pressure; b) processed foods are typically high in sodium; c) fresh, unprocessed food is generally lower in sodium. Answers: b, c.
6. One teaspoon of salt contains: a) 2300 milligrams of sodium; b) more sodium than most adults need in a day; c) the same amount of sodium, regardless of its source. Answer: a, b,c.
7. To keep blood pressure normal, some adults need to limit a) bacon cheeseburgers; b) processed foods; c) prime time television. All are correct.
8. Americans get most (75 percent) of our sodium from a) packaged, processed and restaurant foods; b) salt shakers; c) the salt fairy. Answer: a
9. A diet rich in potassium helps a) blunt the effects of salt on blood pressure; b) reduce the risk of developing kidney stones, c) boost the fruit and vegetable industry. All are correct.
10. The proven "Dietary Approach to Stop Hypertension" is: a) called the DASH diet; b) high in calcium and potassium; c) low in salt. All are correct.

REFLECTION: In 2013, the Institute of Medicine (IOM) issued new guidelines for salt intake, noting no strong rationale for Americans to lower their intake of sodium below 2300 milligrams a day. The current recommendation is for adults to consume no more than 2300 milligrams of sodium a day;

African Americans, people with diabetes, high blood pressure or kidney disease, and those older than 51 years of age are advised to limit their daily sodium intake to 1500 milligrams. Stay tuned for new guidelines expected in 2015.

An interesting fact about how the DASH diet might work to lower blood pressure: Nuts, which are recommended on the DASH eating plan, are rich in magnesium. This mineral increases nitric oxide (NO), a beneficial compound that helps keep the walls of our arteries flexible and healthy.

STEPS TO PREVENT OSTEOPOROSIS

It was the phone call I did not want to get. "Mom's in the emergency room," my sister said. "She fell down the front steps at her house." Thank heaven, aside from a bump on her head and a bruised nose, she didn't break any bones.

My mom has several risk factors for osteoporosis, a disease characterized by weak porous bones. She's female. (Women are five times more susceptible to weakened bones than men.) She is past the age of menopause when bone loss accelerates due to the loss of estrogen. She's Caucasian which puts her at higher risk for developing osteoporosis. (Women of Asian descent are also at higher risk for this disease.)

On the plus side, Mom comes from solid stock; she's not underweight. And she's never struggled with an eating disorder. (Being underweight, weighing less than 127 pounds, or following extremely limited diets can accelerate bone loss.) Fortunately too, Mom has never smoked cigarettes and she drinks alcohol only occasionally. (Smoking and excess alcohol can be toxic to bones.)

Her daughter (yours truly) bugs her frequently to get enough calcium in her diet and supplements to total about 1500 milligrams a day. She does pretty well; she consumes 2 to 3 servings of milk or yogurt most days. (These foods provide about 300 milligrams of calcium per cup.) And the soy beverage she likes is enriched with calcium and vitamin D.

When she takes calcium supplements, Mom takes them in doses of about 500 to 600 milligrams; that's about the maximum amount the body can absorb at one time.

Being from New Mexico, my mom knows that vitamin D, the nutrient that helps her body absorb calcium, is activated when our skin is exposed to sunlight. But her beautiful complexion shows that she doesn't rely on the sun to get adequate vitamin D. I've advised her to consume at least 600 International Units (IU) a day, and more if her doctor advises it. She gets about 100 IU in each cup of milk or fortified soy beverage she consumes; and daily multivitamin contains about 400 IU vitamin D.

Mom's lively little dog Mindy, takes her out for frequent walks to the park, providing weight-bearing exercise that strengthens her bones. Just watch those steps.

CAN DO'S TO LOWER BREAST CANCER RISK

Don't get me wrong. My gynecologist is a great doctor. I just don't consider my annual visit to her office the highlight of my year. And I hold the same sentiment for my yearly mammography appointment. Although a sign in the exam room reassures me that, "We compress because we care," I can still think of other things I would rather do. But I know this is an important choice. And I can make other choices to lessen the threat of breast cancer in my life, say experts:

I can respect real food. While promoters attempt to convince me that various pills and potions are the end-all answer to my nutritional health, I will put my faith in the natural foods of this earth. Foods from the orchard and garden such as fruit, vegetables, and whole grains—supply the most potent cancer-fighting substances known to man.

I can add more vegetables and fruit to my diet. A recent study on women at risk for developing breast cancer concluded, "The protective effect of increased intake of fruits and vegetables is overwhelmingly consistent for breast cancer as well as for most other cancers." This is true not just because vegetables and fruit are rich in beta carotene, vitamin C and other antioxidant nutrients. It's rather the *combination* of these substances in whole foods that exert such a powerful effect against cancer. In fact, studies that have looked for a protective effect of isolated nutrients in supplements against cancer have been less convincing than those which have studied whole foods. By far, the best combination of substances that protect against cancer is found in nature's original packaging.

I can eat less fat. When DNA—the genetic code imbedded in each cell of our bodies—gets damaged, errant cancer cells have a better chance to grow. One study showed that healthy women with a family history of breast cancer who ate less fat in their diets had less damage to their DNA (as measured by a blood test) than women who ate more fat.

I can use my crockpot more often. Meat that is cooked at lower temperatures, such as slow-cooked soups and stews, are less apt to form reactive substances that can damage DNA, say researchers. Meat that is grilled, broiled, roasted or fried at higher temperatures can form substances which become oxidized and damage the genetic code (DNA) in cells. This "oxidative DNA damage" may play a role in the growth and progression of cancerous tumors, say experts.

I can eat beef and pork less often. Some studies have found that the risk for breast cancer increases as the intake of meat (especially red meat) goes up. No such association has been found with poultry or fish.

I don't have to follow a wacky diet. Raw vegetables are great; so are cooked vegetables. Both are protective against breast cancer.

And life is more than a bowl of carrots. Beware of any anti-cancer diet strategy that eliminates major nutrient groups.

REFLECTION: In 2014, the National Cancer Institute (NCI) stated, "It is not proven that a diet low in fat or high in fruits and vegetables will prevent breast cancer." At the same time, this organization reported new evidence that increased plant-based foods (including vegetable oils, nuts, and proteins) and higher intakes of fish oils (omega-3's) decrease the risk for breast cancer. Experts continue to debate whether meat intake is associated with breast cancer risk; some recent studies have failed to show a link.

These lifestyle strategies however, are strong protectors against breast cancer, says the NCI:

- *Maintain a healthy weight, especially after menopause. Extra fat cells produce estrogen, a hormone that feeds a certain type of breast cancer. Interestingly, the risk for breast cancer is higher for women who become overweight as adults; it's also higher for those with "apple" shapes who tend to carry extra pounds around the middle. Apples who are overweight also carry an increased risk for heart disease and type 2 diabetes.*
- *Get in at least 4 hours of exercise each week. Physical activity increases the activity of infection-fighting T-cells and may improve survival in women who go through chemotherapy, according to research conducted at Pennsylvania State University. Exercise also helps decrease hormone levels which lowers the risk for certain types of cancer.*
- *If you drink alcohol, limit your intake to no more than one drink a day. Your risk for breast cancer rises as your intake of alcohol increases.*

Quinn-Essential Nutrition

EAT TO BEAT CANCER

The American Cancer Society calls itself "The official sponsor of birthdays." I like that. It reminds me that we have hope to beat this menacing disease.

What is cancer? It's a term used for more than 100 different diseases with one common theme—uncontrolled growth of abnormal cells in the body. Half of all men and one-third of women in the United States will develop cancer in their lifetimes, says the ACS. That's the bad news; the good news is that one in every three cases of cancer is preventable. And much of what we can do involves the food we choose to eat, according to a recent report from the _World Cancer Research Fund_. Here are some of their current recommendations:

- **Be as lean as possible without becoming underweight.** It's true; any amount of extra weight, especially around the middle, is strongly linked to cancer, especially colon cancer.
- **Be physically active for at least 30 minutes every day.** Exercise helps normalize hormone levels and strengthens our immune system; both are important to beat cancer.
- **Stay away from sugar-sweetened drinks and eat fewer foods that are calorie-rich but nutrient-poor.** Sugar per se does not cause cancer, but too many sugary, high calorie foods can pack on the pounds and increase cancer risk that way, say experts.
- **Fill most of your plate with plant-based foods.** Vegetables and fruit contain a host of substances that protect cells in the body from cancer-causing agents. Whole grains, beans, nuts and other plant foods also contain fiber that keeps food moving through the digestive system and reduces the risk of some types of intestinal cancers.
- **Eat smaller portions of beef, pork and lamb "red meats" and try to avoid processed meats as much as possible.** "Studies show we can eat up to 18 ounces (cooked weight) of red meat a week without raising cancer risk," says the AICR.

This includes beef, lamb and pork. "Research on processed meat (meats preserved by smoking, curing, or salting) shows cancer risk starts to increase with any portion."

Other recommendations: Limit alcohol to no more than 2 drinks a day for men and 1 a day for women. Go easy on salty foods. Feed your newborns breast milk exclusively for at least 6 months. And don't go nuts with high-dose dietary supplements. The best defense against cancer, say experts, is a balanced and varied diet.

REFLECTION: In 2012, a review by the American Institute of Cancer Research (AICR) stated that breast cancer patients and survivors no longer need to worry about eating moderate amounts of soy foods. Results from human studies show that soy consumption does not lead to increased estrogen levels as previously feared. In fact, research on humans showed no increase in any type of cancer from soy foods, according to the AICR. In some cases, the risk for cancer was actually lower due to soy consumption.

What is considered a moderate intake of soy? Most experts agree on 1 or 2 daily servings of whole soy food such as soy beans, tofu, soy milk or edamame. One serving is 1 cup soy milk, ½ cup cooked soy beans, tofu or edamame or ⅓ cup (1 ounce) soy nuts. According to the AICR, no increased risk for breast cancer has been found in even 3 servings of soy foods a day.

BURNING REASONS NOT TO SMOKE

I work in a smoke-free hospital. Signs everywhere remind us that smoking is not permitted anywhere in our facility. If our bodies could post similar signs to remind us not to smoke, this is what they might say:

Caution! Burning inside. Tobacco smoke causes the stomach to produce more acid; it then weakens the pyloric sphincter that normally prevents strong stomach acids from backing up into the esophagus. Result? People who smoke experience more heartburn. And like a cruel joke, heartburn medications do not work as effectively in smokers.

Yield to oncoming bone loss. Smoking causes bones to lose calcium, which may explain why smokers experience more fractured spines, forearms, and hips than non-smokers. A study on Japanese American men found that for every ten years a man smoked, his risk for breaking a bone increased by 10 to 30 percent. And for teens who are still growing, lighting up can burn up any chance for achieving their optimal bone mass.

Stop for heart disease. Nicotine and other by-products of tobacco smoke chemically oxidize dangerous LDL cholesterol in the blood. It's this oxidized LDL that deposits inside artery walls which is one reason why smokers are more at risk for heart attacks and strokes.

Uncontrolled antioxidant burn. Smoking increases the body's need for valuable antioxidant nutrients like vitamins C, E, and beta carotene; they mop up dangerous free radicals that form more readily in people who smoke. When the body depletes its supply of antioxidants, free radicals are set loose to cause damage, resulting in premature aging, cataracts, cancer, or heart disease. Supplemental doses of vitamin C may alleviate some of the damage; however, there is evidence that vitamin E and beta carotene supplements are not helpful and may even be harmful for people who smoke.

Watch for falling hormones. Women who smoke can expect to go through menopause an average of one to two years earlier than non-smokers. That means they lose the health-protective effects of the hormone estrogen sooner than their non-smoking friends. Men who smoke tend to have a higher incidence of impotence than those who do not.

Danger! Cancer Ahead. Even smokeless tobacco harbors cancer-causing chemicals. And although fruits and vegetables contain substances that can inhibit the growth of cancer cells, experts say all bets are off for smokers. Folate for example, is a vitamin found in fruits and vegetables that may reduce the risk for colon cancer. Yet smoking impairs the beneficial effects of this nutrient.

Thank you for not smoking. Besides cooking up blackened lungs, the 4000 or so chemicals in cigarette and cigar smoke do serious damage to the body's ability to process nutrients. Reach for a carrot instead; it's better for your breath and won't stain your teeth.

FORMULA FOR BRIGHT EYES

"The eye is the lamp of the body. If your eyes are healthy, your whole body will be full of light." So goes a verse from the book of Matthew. It's true. Our view of the world comes through light that is filtered and focused through our eyes. And clear vision comes through eyes that are healthy and well-nourished.

Case in point: A landmark study in 2001 sponsored by the *Eye Institute of the National Institutes of Health* found that a specific formula of nutrients and antioxidants significantly reduced the risk of age-related macular degeneration (AMD) in adults at risk for this disease. AMD is the main cause of blindness in adults over age 55, according to the American Optometric Association www.aoa.org.

Volunteers in this study which was dubbed the "Age-Related Eye Disease Study" or AREDS, benefited from a daily supplement that contained vitamin C, vitamin E, beta carotene, zinc, and copper. In 2013, the same team of researchers conducted a second study, AREDS2, to determine if the original AREDS formula could or should be improved for people at risk for eye disease.

One major finding from this latest study: Lutein and zeaxanthin, protective carotenoid substances in plants, were safe

Quinn-Essential Nutrition

and effective substitutes for beta carotene, the carotenoid used in the first AREDS study. This was goods news since former smokers who took beta carotene in the original study had a higher incidence of lung cancer. Based on the promising results of this research, AREDS2 formulas are now hitting the dietary supplement market.

Here are the details from the American Optometric Association:

Lutein (LOO-teen) and zeaxanthin (zee-a-ZAN-thin) belong to the family of carotenoid substances in plant foods that help protect the macula of the eye from harmful rays of light. (The macula is the region of the eye that helps us see fine details.) Found abundantly in green leafy vegetables, these two powerful antioxidants have been shown to reduce the risk of chronic eye diseases such as age-related macular degeneration (AMD) and cataracts. In the AREDS studies, supplements containing 10 milligrams (mg) of lutein and 2 mg of zeaxanthin were beneficial to eye health.

Vitamin C is a powerful antioxidant that promotes the health of blood vessels in the eye. Vitamin C has also been found to lower the risk for developing cataracts, a condition which causes the clear lens of the eyes to become clouded and blur vision. The amount of vitamin C in the AREDS formula was 500 milligrams, higher than the current recommended daily intake (RDI) of 90 mg for men and 75 mg for women.

Vitamin E is a strong antioxidant that protects and keeps the eye in good repair. This nutrient has also been shown to reduce the formation of cataracts and the progression of age-related macular degeneration (AMD). A daily supplement that contained 400 International Units (IU) of vitamin E benefited eye health in the AREDS study.

Zinc is an essential mineral that protects the eye from the formation of cataracts. A deficiency of zinc can impair vision, especially night vision. Found in foods such as beans, nuts, seafood, and whole grains, the AREDS2 formula contains 25 milligrams of zinc. And because zinc can interfere with the absorption of copper, the AREDS formula contains an addition of 2 milligrams copper.

Omega-3 fatty acids, docosahexaenoic acid (thankfully abbreviated DHA) and eicosapentaenoic acid (EPA) are vital components within the retina of the eye. Primarily found in fatty fish, omega-3's are essential for normal eye development during pregnancy and in growing children. In adults, low levels of omega-3 fats have been linked to dry eye syndrome and other serious eye diseases including retinopathy which affects the retina (the seeing part of the eye) and age-related macular degeneration (AMD). Omega 3 fats were not included in the original AREDS formula. But curiously, the addition of 1000 milligrams (1 gram) of omega-3's to the AREDS2 formula resulted in no additional benefit for people with advanced age-related eye disease.

Experts tell us the very best way to nourish our eyes is to eat a varied diet rich in all these essential nutrients. If you've got some nutritional gaps, consider adding a daily multivitamin/mineral supplement. And talk to your doctor or eye professional about the possible benefits of an AREDS or AREDS2 formula.

REFLECTION: While the AREDS studies showed a benefit to eye health with a supplement that included 400 IU vitamin E, another well-executed randomized placebo-controlled trial, the Selenium and Vitamin E Cancer Prevention Trial (SELECT), found an increased risk for prostate cancer in a subset of men who took 400 IU of vitamin E as an individual supplement.

Confusing, yes, but it also reminds us of the strong synergy at work when we consume nutrients in foods rather than isolated in supplements. Concentrated doses of vitamin E may yield unwanted results; yet the health effects of consuming vitamin E-rich foods such as almonds, sunflower seeds, peanuts, and whole grains is beneficial.

DIRTY DOZEN IN PERSPECTIVE

I gulped down a handful of juicy red grapes as we ran out the door. My friend Chris munched on an apple as we drove out of town. Later we ate some strawberries. Should we worry? According to the Environmental Working Group, a nonprofit organization whose stated mission is "to protect public health and the environment," these foods are targeted on a scary-sounding list called the "Dirty Dozen." Foods on this list have higher levels of pesticide residues, says the EWG. Buy the organic version of these products, they advise.

Not so fast, says the Alliance for Food and Farming, another nonprofit that represents farmers of organic and conventional crops. This organization believes the conclusions reached by the EWG may unnecessarily scare people from eating perfectly safe and healthy food.

The issue, says food toxicologist, Carl Winter from the University of California at Davis, stems from the methods used by the EWG to come up with their Dirty Dozen list. It's not just the presence of residues on a food that determines risk, says Winter. It's the amount. His research on these same crops—organic as well as conventionally grown—found the potential risk from exposure to pesticides was negligible. To put it in perspective, the Alliance for Food and Farming estimates that if, in one day, a child ate 154 conventionally grown apples with the highest pesticide residue ever recorded, he or she would still not ingest a level found to have an effect on health.

The main point is not whether a crop is grown with the use of organic or conventional pesticides, but whether or not we are eating those foods. Truckloads of studies over the past decades show without a doubt that eating fruits and vegetables have definite health benefits. And most of these studies were conducted with conventional crops. Whether we choose organic *or* conventionally grown crops, we can lower our risk of dying too soon by eating seven or more servings of fruits and vegetables each day. (A serving is about ½ cup cooked or 1 cup raw fruit or vegetable.)

Even the authors of the Dirty Dozen list confirmed, "The health benefits of a diet rich in fruits and vegetables outweigh risks of pesticide exposure." As one expert said, we should all try to minimize the amount of pesticides on the food we eat. But we don't have to avoid conventionally produced foods to meet that goal.

NUTRITION SOLUTIONS

UNDERSTANDING FOOD ALLERGIES

Don't take food allergies lightly. Although many reactions to food are not life threatening, some are for some people. In fact, more than a hundred susceptible Americans die each year after eating nuts or peanuts, according to Dr. Chad Oh, immunologist at the University of California Los Angeles (UCLA) and author of *How to Live with a Nut Allergy*. Take this quiz to see what you know about food allergies:

1. All of these are common food allergens except: a) fish; b) wheat and eggs; c) coconut; d) milk and soy; e) peanuts and tree nuts. Answer: c.
2. Symptoms related to food allergies include: a) skin rashes; b) wheezing; c) sneezing; d) swollen lips. All are correct.
3. How soon after eating can symptoms of food allergy develop? a) within minutes; b) within hours; c) between commercials. All are correct; reaction times vary with each individual.
4. The culprit in food that initiates an allergic response is a) fat; b) carbohydrate; c) protein; d) Donald Trump. Answer: c.
5. A reliable way to diagnose a food allergy is: a) ask your hairdresser; b) see a board certified allergist; c) participate in a double-blind placebo-controlled food challenge (DBPCFC). Answers: b, c. Other tests may help identify

food allergies but the most reliable is a food "challenge" by a trained immunologist.
6. An effective way to manage a confirmed food allergy is to: a) order mega doses of vitamins off the internet; b) ignore it and maybe it will go away; c) avoid the offending food. Answer: c.
7. An "elimination diet" is a) high in fiber to help you eliminate better; b) eliminates all foods that may cause an allergic reaction; c) may be deficient in essential nutrients. Answers: b, c
8. True or False? Food allergies are the same as food intolerances. False. Allergies involve the immune system and are usually caused by specific proteins in food. Intolerances can be triggered by other substances in food; an intolerance to lactose, the sugar in milk, is one example.
9. What percentage of people allergic to peanuts (a legume), are also allergic to tree nuts such as walnuts and pecans? a) 50 percent; b) 10 percent; c) repeat the question, please. Answer: a.
10. Women who are at high risk for food allergies may be able to lower their infant's risk for allergies if they: a) breastfeed; b) eat foods rich in vitamin C during lactation; c) stay away from chocolate-covered peanuts. Answer: a,b,c. A 2005 study in Finland concluded that a woman's diet during lactation that is rich in natural sources of vitamin C (not supplements) might reduce the risk for allergies in high risk infants. And the *American Academy of Pediatrics* recommends that breastfeeding women at high risk for allergies avoid peanut and tree nuts to decrease their infant's risk for severe food allergies.
11. Severe food allergies a) may get worse with each exposure; b) are often not related to the amount of food eaten; c) can be life threatening. All are correct.
12. If you have a severe allergy to nuts, you should: a) not take a peanut flight; b) avoid even small traces of nuts; c) wear a Medic Alert bracelet. All are correct.

Quinn-Essential Nutrition

> REFLECTION: *Findings from the largest study on this topic to date were published in the Annals of Allergy, Asthma and Clinical Immunology in July, 2013. Here are their key findings:*
>
> - *About a fourth of the children (26 percent) outgrew their food allergies around the age of 5 years.*
> - *Children were most likely to outgrow allergies to milk, egg, or soy. They were less likely to outgrow allergies to shellfish, tree nuts, and peanuts.*
> - *Children who were younger in age when they had their first reaction to a food were more likely to outgrow the allergy.*

DIET TO EASE SORE JOINTS

So my doggie comes back from vacation all puffed and fluffed, nails trimmed and teeth cleaned. Nice to have a veterinarian for a son-in-law. My dog also has a new diagnosis, degenerative joint disease (DJD). Will is an active dog; he's had lots of wear and tear on his joints these eight years of his doggie life. But he sure seems too young to be suffering with this.

"Could be genetic…or nutritional," Dr. Tom informs me. So he sends us home with a prescription dog food especially formulated for Will's joint disease. And of course I check out the ingredients:

Omega-3 fatty acids. These fats are essential for humans, but can they preserve cartilage in Will's joints? One recent study in the *Journal of the American Veterinary Medical Association* found that dogs with osteoarthritis (another word for degenerative joint disease) were better able to move, walk and play when they were fed food with high levels of omega-3 fatty acids. Human studies on the effects of increased omega-3's for degenerative joint disease are less clear, but promising, say experts.

Antioxidants. Will's dog food contains "clinically proven antioxidants to support healthy immune function." Makes sense. In humans with osteoarthritis, scientists have observed excessive numbers of "radical oxygen species," molecules that damage body tissues. Antioxidant nutrients like vitamin C, vitamin E and selenium scavenge the body for these harmful molecules and render them harmless. Vitamin C is also used to make collagen, an essential component of connective tissue to hold Will's joints together when he chases deer out of the yard. Vitamin C also helps the body manufacture a protein-like compound called *L-carnitine* which helps transport toxic compounds out of active muscle cells.

Selenium is another antioxidant nutrient that can neutralize harmful free radicals and relieve symptoms of arthritis, according to the US Office of Dietary Supplements. Selenium is found naturally in foods such as beef, tuna and Brazil nuts.

Glucosamine and chondroitin. These compounds help cartilage, the body's connective tissue, absorb water and thereby keep joints lubricated. One of the largest studies to look at the effectiveness of these substances on joint health was the Glucosamine/chondroitin Arthritis Intervention Trial (GAIT). Results from this large clinical trial that tested the effects of glucosamine hydrochloride (glucosamine) and sodium chondroitin sulfate (chondroitin sulfate) for the treatment of knee osteoarthritis—found no significant differences in pain relief between these supplements and Celebrex (a non-steroidal anti-inflammatory drug (NSAID).

However, one subset of patients with moderate to severe knee pain did report significant pain relief on a combination of 1500 milligrams glucosamine (500 mg three times a day) plus 1200 mg chondroitin sulfate (400 mg three times a day). Because of the small size of this subgroup, these researchers consider these findings preliminary.

In addition to his special diet, Dr. Tom gave Will a prescription injection of selenium and vitamin E and cautioned me about possible side effects; another reminder that even nutrition interventions need to be monitored closely.

Back home, Will's diet was pretty easy; everything he needed was in one bag. Meals are a bit more complicated for us humans. Experts tell us the best "anti-inflammation" diet is one that includes sources of omega-three fatty acids such as fish, flax and walnuts and high doses of antioxidant nutrients such as fruits, vegetables, and whole grains.

Alas, dogs are not humans and humans are not dogs. So it's always a good idea to consult the expert of your particular species. Thanks, Dr. Tom!

GOUT: TALE OF THE ACHING TOE

Once upon a time there lived a wealthy king. Each time he returned victorious from battle, he would declare a celebration feast of rich meats, gravies, and strong ale. And the more the great king succeeded, the more he would feast and imbibe. One day as the king pushed away from his banquet table, he experienced a sharp pain in his toe that continued up his leg.

"Ouch!" he bellowed. He immediately called for the royal physician and the royal dietitian. After much examination, they determined that indeed, the king suffered from gout, one of the oldest diseases in recorded history.

"Why do I have such pain?" asked the king.

"Because, your Highness," the physician explained, "your blood contains high amounts of uric acid. This chemical turns into crystals that have accumulated in your joints. The pain you feel is an inflammatory condition which will be called 'arthritis' in a few hundred years."

The king turned to the royal dietitian. "What can I do to avoid this misery?"

"You must change your ways, oh king," said the wise dietitian. "Many of your favorite foods, such as liver and other organ meats, sardines, and anchovies, contain high levels of proteins called 'purines.' These turn into uric acid, the substance that is causing you pain."

"Must I give up *all* my favorite feasts?" the king cried.

"You must learn to eat smaller portions of high protein animal foods," the dietitian replied. She pointed to the king's servants. "Your humble subjects subsist on cereals, fruits and vegetables… and they rarely suffer with gout."

The king frowned. "And my ale? Must I give it up as well?"

"Too much will certainly cause you pain," she said.

"What else can be done to relieve my suffering?" the king asked.

"Call for the royal pharmacist," answered the physician. "He will prepare a medicine to lower the uric acid in your blood. And your highness would be wise to lose a few pounds."

"I shall lose some weight in a hurry with a low-carbohydrate diet!" declared the king.

"I would humbly advise you to retain carbohydrate foods such as grains, fruit, and vegetables at your banquet table," said the royal dietitian. "And if you eat less meat and gravy, this will lessen your risk for another painful attack."

The king whimpered, "And water instead of ale, I suppose?"

"At least a liter of water a day, your excellence," said the royal physician.

And so the king took the counsel of the royal health team and he lived happily ever after.

DIET TO FIGHT YEAST INFECTIONS

"I struggle with reoccurring yeast infections," a reader writes. "The doctor gave me an oral medication and I didn't have infections for a year. Then my body became allergic to the medicine. I know I can change my diet, but you know how hard that is! I know I need to cut out refined sugar and starches. Again not so easy! Can you give me some ideas to eat for breakfast? It's hard to go to the store with four kids and actually read the labels."

Dear Reader,

You'll find a lot of fascinating information about this condition, but not much that's reliable. Suffice it to say, some diet changes can help prevent yeast infections. But it may not be as drastic as you have been led to believe. Here's why:

Yeasts are everywhere. They live in soil; they reside on the skins of fruit and berries; and they live in the body. Some yeasts are good and others are not. The yeast most often responsible for infections in the body is *Candida albicans*. Although always present, *Candida* is considered an "opportunistic pathogen:" it is only harmful if it grows out of control.

What's the most common cause of yeast infections? Antibiotic use, say experts. When we take antibiotics to treat an illness, good bacteria that protect the body from yeast overgrowth are destroyed along with bad bacteria. Other conditions that promote the abnormal growth of yeast in the body include pregnancy, hormone replacement therapy, diabetes and HIV infections.

Yeasts in food are entirely different species from the pathogen *Candida albicans*, however. Like edible mushrooms, nutritional yeasts are considered "friendly fungi." *Saccharomyces cerevisiae*, for example, is a common yeast used to make bread. Other strains of *Saccharomyces* ferment grape juice into wine. Kombucha, a fermented sweet tea, is made with a nutritional yeast. Some yeasts are even used to turn corn into ethanol fuel. But I digress.

You can find all kinds of advice on how to prevent yeast infections. One internet site says you must eliminate everything but garlic, spices, herbs and vegetables. Here are some reliable remedies:

Increase your intake of *Lactobacillus acidophilus* (*L. acidophilus*). These good bacteria prevent *Candida* yeast cells from growing out of control. And as hard as it is to read food labels with four kids in tow, check to see that these good bacteria are in the milk, kefir, or yogurt you buy.

Keep up your defenses. Protein-type foods strengthen your immune system and push back the growth of wayward yeast cells.

Include a source of protein such as fish, poultry, meat, eggs, low-fat cheese, yogurt, milk, beans, or nuts with every meal.

Make half your plate vegetables. Cooked or raw, these foods feed the beneficial bacteria in the gut to keep the bad *Candida* boys under control.

Add some raw garlic. Garlic has proven anti-fungal and anti-bacterial properties. Smash raw cloves and add them to salad dressings or other fresh foods.

Consider taking a probiotic supplement. Probiotics such as *Lactobacillus* are good bacteria that can control the growth of *Candida*. One trustworthy brand is Culturelle® which contains *Lactobacillus GG*.

Cut out extra sugar, including juice and sugared beverages. Choose whole fruit instead.

And here's an idea for breakfast: Scoop plain or low-sugar yogurt made with *Lactobacillus* "live active" cultures into a bowl; then sprinkle with some raw garlic…just kidding.

Most importantly, avoid the overuse of antibiotics. Let your doctor know about your symptoms so she can prescribe necessary medical therapy. And don't believe everything you read on the internet.

HEALING BROKEN BONES

Rule No. 1: When you get bucked off your horse, try to land on your feet.

Rule No.2: Don't break anything when you land.

"I have good news and bad news," my doctor told me. "The bad news is you have a broken bone in your foot." And the good news?

"It's a stable break that won't require surgery. Should be healed in two to four weeks...if you take care of it."

Gee, that's nice. So what does my broken bone need in order to heal? This is what I learned:

Stability. I promise to be good and wear my protective boot splint and use my crutches as instructed.

Good circulation. Blood flow carries healing oxygen, nutrients, and cellular building blocks to connect and heal broken tissue. This process is called "remodeling."

Nutrition. Much of the "glue" that mends broken bones is found in food. Protein helps manufacture collagen that knits bones back together. Primary sources of protein include eggs, meat, fish, poultry, nuts, soy, and dairy foods. Smaller amounts of protein are found in grains and vegetables. Vitamin C is essential for collagen formation as well. Foods high in vitamin C include peppers, strawberries, broccoli, tomatoes, oranges and grapefruit.

Calcium is the primary mineral in bone tissue and we need vitamin D to absorb calcium. Milk is a good source of both these nutrients as well as valuable protein. Other good options are calcium and vitamin D enriched soy beverages.

Vitamin K helps to pack strengthening minerals into my bones. I will remember to eat more leafy greens like kale, Swiss chard and spinach; all are excellent sources of vitamin K.

Even when I do what my doc tells me, some bones just naturally heal faster than others. Bones in the toes, for example, tend to heal quickly because they are fairly stable and receive a good supply of healing blood. Bones in the wrist have a more limited blood supply and may take longer to heal, say experts.

"Do you want a prescription for pain medication?" my emergency room doctor asked me. I declined but later took a mild pain reliever at home when I needed it. Best not to overuse these meds, I learned. Medications that reduce pain and inflammation can actually slow down the healing process if we rely on them too much. Through the pain, my body produces chemicals that begin the process of repairing my broken bone. The release of these chemicals is blocked if I rely too heavily on anti-inflammatory medicines like aspirin and ibuprofen.

I was happy to learn that, once a bone completes the healing process, it is totally restored. "The healed area is brand new, without a scar. Usually thicker, the new bone may even be stronger than the old," says Martin Yahiro, M.D., a Baltimore orthopedist and consultant to the Food and Drug Administration.

REFLECTION: Although the minerals calcium and phosphorous make up at least half the volume of bones, the other half is protein. Recent studies have shown that diets high in protein as well as calcium are beneficial for bone health.

CELIAC DISEASE AND GLUTEN

Celiac disease is also called celiac sprue or gluten intolerance. Here are some other facts about this condition:

Celiac disease is different from an allergy to wheat. It is an intolerance to gluten, a protein in wheat, rye, and barley grains. Considered an autoimmune disease, gluten sets off an immune reaction that triggers an attack on the small intestine. In the process, the nutrient-absorbing surface of the digestive tract is destroyed. This can lead to severe deficiencies of key nutrients such as iron, folate, calcium, vitamins A, D, E and K.

Celiac has been estimated to affect 1 in 133 people in the United States, and most of these remain undiagnosed, according to the National Foundation for Celiac Awareness (NFCA). Women are two to threes times more likely to have celiac disease than men. And since it is an autoimmune disorder, people with other autoimmune conditions (such as type 1 diabetes) have a higher risk to develop celiac disease.

Interestingly, celiac is less common in individuals who were breastfed as babies and were not fed gluten-containing foods such as wheat, rye or barley cereals before the age of four months.

Celiac is often difficult to diagnose. Common symptoms include stomach pain, bloating, diarrhea, constipation, and poor appetite. It is best diagnosed with a biopsy, a sample of tissue snipped from the small intestine and examined for signs of damage. Blood tests are also being refined to better identify celiac disease. Once diagnosed, celiac is effectively treated with a strict gluten-free diet for life.

Gluten is a protein compound found in wheat, rye and barley grains. It is not naturally found in oats. However, oats might contain traces of wheat if both these grains are processed in the same facility.

Other gluten-containing grains include spelt (an ancient species of wheat), triticale (a hybrid grain of wheat and rye) and couscous (granules of durum wheat). Be cautious too, of foods labeled "wheat-free" which might contain gluten from rye or barley.

Gluten is *not* found in flax, quinoa, potato, rice or corn. Fruit and vegetables and their juices are also naturally free of gluten. Wine is considered a gluten-free food but it might be present in beer brewed with barley.

Nutrition therapy aimed to avoid all sources of gluten in the diet is the only proven and effective treatment for celiac disease.

Barbara A. Quinn, MS, RD, CDE

> REFLECTION: Research continues to refine the diagnosis and treatment of celiac disease. Blood tests in particular have been refined to better diagnose this disorder, according to the National Digestive Diseases Information Clearinghouse (NDDIC). Labs can now identify high levels of anti-tissue transglutaminase antibodies (tTGA) and anti-endomysium antibodies (EMA) to help to identify celiac disease.
>
> Hurray, too, that in 2013, the United States Food and Drug Administration (FDA) formally defined the term "gluten-free" for food products. In line with standards set by the World Health Organization, the European Union and Canada, a food is considered gluten-free if it contains less than 20 parts per million (ppm) of any gluten-containing substance. Read on...

GLUTEN-FREE DEFINED AT LAST

My younger daughter and I joke that her future wedding song, when Mr. Right finally comes along, will be Celine Dion's rendition of "At Last." We might want to sing the same about the much-anticipated definition of the term "gluten-free" by the US Food and Drug Administration (FDA). At last, we have the official description of "gluten-free" food in accordance with the 2004 Food Allergen Labeling and Consumer Protection Act.

What's the big deal? Celiac disease, an autoimmune disorder which requires the strict avoidance of gluten, affects an estimated three million Americans. (Gluten is a composite of proteins that occur naturally in wheat, rye and barley grains.) And some people are sensitive to gluten even without a clear diagnosis of celiac disease.

One thing the FDA is clear about: A food labeled "gluten-free" cannot contain any wheat, rye, barley or mixtures of these grains.

Any incidental gluten in a food must be less than 20 parts per million (ppm) in order to carry the gluten-free label.

Why not zero gluten instead of the allowed 20 ppm? Two reasons, says the FDA. No scientifically validated method exists that can reliably detect gluten at a level lower than 20 parts per million. And research suggests that most individuals with celiac disease can tolerate occasional trace amounts of gluten (less than 20 ppm) with no adverse effects.

Use of the "gluten-free" term is voluntary; a food that is gluten-free does not have to say so on the label. Bottled water, for example, is not required to display a gluten-free label unless the manufacturer so chooses. Any food that makes the gluten-free claim, however, must abide by the FDA's definition. Meats, poultry, some egg products and alcohol are excluded from this rule however, since they are not regulated by the FDA.

REFLECTION: Celiac disease remains tricky to diagnose. Some people present with classic symptoms such as diarrhea, bloating, and abdominal pain. Others do not. Other symptoms which may or may not point to celiac include anemia, bone loss, migraine headaches, and liver abnormalities. The term "silent" celiac disease is sometimes used to describe less common presentations of this disorder.

Since celiac is an autoimmune disease, people with other autoimmune disorders such as rheumatoid arthritis, Addison's disease, and Sjogren's syndrome should be tested for this condition. And people with type 1 diabetes should also be screened, according to guidelines by the American Diabetes Association.

Barbara A. Quinn, MS, RD, CDE

OVERCOMING BAD BUGS WITH GOOD

It's spooky to think that good and bad are fighting it out inside us every day. And with an estimated 100 trillion bacterial cells in the human intestinal tract, let's pray the good side wins.

Like an old Clint Eastwood flick, the flora that grows in our lower intestines is combination of good, bad and ugly microbes. Beneficial bacteria such as *Lactobacillus* and *Bifidobacterium* help manufacture vitamin K, fortify our immune system, and prevent the growth of harmful bacteria such as the notorious *E.coli*. Things get ugly when this balance is disturbed.

Research shows that an imbalance of "bowel flora" may play a role in the development of allergies, especially during infancy. And breastfed babies tend to have a more healthful balance of gut bacteria than formula-fed babies. Other studies have found that inflammatory bowel diseases such as ulcerative colitis, Crohn's disease and irritable bowel syndrome (IBS) may be linked to an unhealthy balance of intestinal bacteria.

Where do we find beneficial bacteria and how do we encourage their proliferation? Check the next carton of yogurt you buy for the words "live and active cultures." These are the good microbes (probiotics) used to make yogurt, kefir, and other fermented foods; common names include *Lactobacillus acidophilus, S.thermohilus, L. bulgaris* and *bifidus*.

Just like yeast needs a little sugar to grow, probiotics need "prebiotics" to thrive. Prebiotics are therefore the food for probiotics that reside in the fibers of plant foods such as fruit, vegetables and whole grains. Inulin and oligofructose for example, occur naturally in a long list of foods including oatmeal, flax, barley and other whole grains, onions, greens such as dandelion, spinach, collard, chard, kale and mustard greens, berries, bananas, lentils, kidney beans and other legumes.

What kind and how much of these prebiotics and probiotics do we need? Ah, that is the question. Scientists are just beginning to understand all the complexities of these healthy intestinal flora. Like planting a garden, our guts tend to produce the bacteria we sow.

A bed of beneficial bacteria takes root when we plant food sources of probiotics (yogurt and other fermented foods) and feed them with a healthful mix of prebiotics from fruit, vegetables and whole grains. When the good outweighs the bad, we can harvest better health. And so the battle rages; and the good guys win in the end.

DIETARY SOLUTIONS FOR DIVERTICULITIS

Once in a very refined land, there lived a man who enjoyed very refined food. He dined on the crispiest, creamiest donuts, the finest coffee, and the most exquisite meats and cheeses. Yet, those around him realized something was missing.

"You need more fiber," his less refined wife said to him. But the man did not understand. Then one day he had severe pain and nausea. He went to his doctor who ordered some tests.

"You have diverticulitis," his doctor told him. But the man did not understand. "Inside your large intestine are weakened areas that bulge out, making little pouches called 'diverticula,'" his doctor explained. "The presence of these little sacs is called 'diverticulosis.' If these little pouches become inflamed or infected, you have 'diverticulitis.'"

"How did this happen to me?" the man asked.

"Good question," said the wise doctor. "Diverticula are little pouches that can form from high pressure inside the large intestine. Diverticular disease is fairly common in the United States and Europe; but it is rare in Africa and Asia where the typical diet is higher in fiber."

The man glanced at his wife. She smiled.

"Can you help me, Doc?" the man pleaded.

"Take these antibiotics," the doctor ordered. And until the infection clears, drink fluids and only eat soft foods that are low in fiber such as white bread, refined cereals, rice, pasta, meat, poultry, fish, dairy foods, juices or soft fruits and vegetables with no seeds or skins. When you are well again, gradually increase your intake of dietary fiber to 25 to 35 grams of fiber a day."

The man was confused so he called his personal dietitian. "How do I eat more fiber?"

"Think plants," she explained. "Fiber is only found in plant-based foods like fruits, vegetables, grains, nuts, and seeds. Fiber adds bulk to your stool and helps ease the passage of waste material through your digestive tract. Most experts believe that a diet high in fiber can help prevent another attack of diverticulitis."

Obviously still confused, the man asked, "How much fiber in a steak?"

"Zero," said the dietitian patiently. "Animal foods do not contain dietary fiber. A piece of fruit, however, contains about 3 grams as does a slice of whole grain bread. And a cup of your favorite cooked beans contains 15 grams of dietary fiber!"

The man frowned. "Anything else I need to know?"

"Daily physical activity and drinking extra water helps move everything to its proper...end," she said gently.

"What about foods with nuts and seeds? Can I still eat these?" he asked.

"Many experts say this restriction is an old wives' tale," the dietitian explained. "But most patients know what gives them distress. Best advice is to chew your food well and be cautious with nuts and tough-skinned foods like corn on the cob. And if you know which foods bother you, don't eat them."

The man took his doctor's advice and followed his dietitian's guidance. He added whole grains, fruit, vegetables and beans to his meals. He became less refined. And then he understood.

REFLECTION: New studies have challenged the view that a low fiber diet increases the risk for diverticulitis. Other factors like age and obesity seem to be involved, say experts. Nevertheless, evidence continues to support the current nutritional treatment for diverticulitis: A low fiber diet low until symptoms subside; then gradually increase your intake of dietary fiber to the daily recommendation of 25 to 35 grams per day.

DIET-BLADDER-PAIN CONNECTION

A reader reminded me that September was "Interstitial Cystitis Awareness" Month. Say again? That's the point, say experts. Interstitial Cystitis (IC) is a condition with which "millions suffer and few understand." Let's try to understand.

According to the *National Institute of Diabetes and Digestive and Kidney Diseases,* IC is "a condition that causes discomfort or pain in the bladder and a need to urinate frequently and urgently." And at the risk of TMI (too much information), interstitial cystitis is also known as bladder pain syndrome or BPS.

This condition is more common in women than in men. And it can be tricky to diagnose since its symptoms are similar to a bladder infection, although IC is not an infection. And it can be tricky to treat as well.

What does this have to do with nutrition? Experts have observed that certain foods may trigger unfortunate symptoms in some people with IC. And while there is no specific diet to treat IC, some sufferers report certain foods to be more abrasive to the bladder than others. Foods most commonly reported to be bothersome for people with IC include alcohol, artificial sweeteners such as aspartame and saccharine, coffee (even decaf in some people), citrus and cranberry juices, hot peppers, carbonated soda, and spicy foods. Others add chocolate, tea and tomatoes to their list of irritating foods.

Not everyone has problems with these foods, however. One way to find out is an elimination diet in which you delete, for at least a month, any food you suspect to be a potential problem. Then one by one, over a period of several weeks, add these foods back into your diet. As you do this, keep track of the foods that worsen your symptoms.

The goal, say experts, is to find the foods you can eat comfortably, not to make yourself miserable. Most patients with IC have a small list of "do not's" and a bigger list of "usually OK" foods based on their symptoms. The best diet to relieve the painful symptoms of interstitial cystitis is one that includes a balanced variety of foods and essential nutrients.

Barbara A. Quinn, MS, RD, CDE

"We do not know exactly why some foods bother most IC patients and other foods do not," says registered dietitian Julie Beyer, MA, RD of the Interstitial Cystitis Association. "The diet-IC connection becomes even more mystifying when we observe that certain foods that bother one patient do not bother others." The good news, she says, is that researchers are taking a closer look at the treatments we have for IC, including nutrition therapies.

WEIGHTY ISSUES

▬▬▬▬▬▬▬▬▬▬ THINK HEALTH NOT WEIGHT

"But I'm too fat to be this healthy!" That was the surprised response from a portly client after I informed him that his cholesterol and other nutritional lab tests were absolutely normal. He had been large all his life, he told me, and had never been successful with long term weight loss. Brings up a good question: Does carrying around extra body weight always add up to poor health? Or to put it another way, if we are overweight, must we assume that we can't be healthy unless we lose weight? The answer is maybe...and maybe not. Here are the reasons for both sides:

Obesity is related to at least half of the main killer diseases in the United States, including heart disease and diabetes. Losing excess poundage often improves these conditions. Yet the continuous cycle of losing weight and gaining it back may damage health more than not losing it in the first place.

Overly strict or unwise diet practices cause the body to lose significant amounts of muscle tissue as well as fat. When muscle, which burns the bulk of our daily calories, is depleted, it's easier to regain weight. And the pounds that come back tend to be fat, not muscle. That's why each cycle of weight loss and weight gain can actually makes us fatter, experts explain.

Another reason to focus on healthful habits more than the weight scale is that our tendency to be round or plump is at least partially inherited. (We can blame our parents.) Case in point:

Scientists have developed a breed of genetically obese rats that are heavy at birth and remain so even when they are fed the same amount of food as normal weight rats. When these fat rats are put on calorie-restricted diets, their growth is stunted but they remain overweight.

Humans are not rats; yet some experts now view obesity as a storage disease that causes an overweight person to store extra calories in their fat cells much more efficiently than a thin person. So what is a genetically overweight yo-yo dieter to do? Maybe it's time to stop being "on" or "off" a diet; focus instead on making better food and exercise choices. Here are some ideas to chew on:

- Accept your God-given body build. And take care of it. Any body type can become strong, vigorous, and attractive with the right combination of nourishing foods and physical activity.
- Understand that being overweight is a chronic condition that you can manage but not entirely cure. No, it is not fair that some people will never have weight issues. But if you do, realize the choices you can make to impact your health.
- Get moving! Vigorous activity for more than 15 minutes at a time forces the body to dip into fat stores for energy. And at least 3 hours of physical exercise each week maintains important muscle mass and strength. Isn't that want we want after all?

REFLECTION: In 2013, the American Medical Association (AMA) voted to officially classify obesity as "a disease state with multiple pathophysiological aspects requiring a range of interventions." Many believe this was a major step to move obesity treatments from stigma to solutions.

Quinn-Essential Nutrition

WHAT'S NOT TRUE ABOUT WEIGHT LOSS PRODUCTS

Some statements don't sound quite right. "Kids Make Good Snacks," for example. Some may be interpreted wrong, such as "Weight Loss Study Looks for Larger Test Group." Others can be downright deceptive, especially when it comes to the selling of products marketed for weight loss.

Let's face it. We are a culture desperate to lose weight. And that makes the sale of weight loss products extremely profitable, even if the claims for their effectiveness are bogus.

To the rescue comes the Federal Trade Commission (FTC) whose job is to protect us from companies that sell products with false or misleading advertising. This agency can help us decide between "Here's my credit card!" and "You've got to be kidding." For example, the FTC says these claims for over-the-counter weight loss products can simply not be true:

Lose 10 pounds every week! Guaranteed! Tilt. Any ad that promises fast and continuous weight loss of more than two pounds a week for a month or more, without serious dieting or exercise, is false, says the FTC.

Lose weight without depriving yourself! If only...but not true, say experts. It is impossible to eat unlimited amounts of any food and still lose weight.

Use this product for six months and get the weight off for good! Uh, no. Keeping weight off for good requires keeping on track with diet and exercise goals...for good.

Just take this pill! No over-the-counter product can block enough fat or calories to lose a large amount of weight, says registered dietitian nutritionist Eleese Cunningham in a recent article in the *Journal of the Academy of Nutrition and Dietetics*. Even legitimate weight loss drugs are only useful when accompanied by a low-calorie diet and exercise.

Barbara A. Quinn, MS, RD, CDE

Safely lose 30 pounds in 30 days! Quick weight loss—more than three pounds a week over multiple weeks—can be risky without medical supervision. Products that promise lightning-fast weight loss are a scam at best, says the FTC. At worst, they can ruin your health.

Works for everybody! Really? Like shoes, no one diet fits everyone. Current research confirms that diets need to be individualized to our unique health and calorie needs.

Simply rub on this miracle diet cream and watch the pounds melt away! You might watch the pounds melt from your wallet but not from your body, says the FTC. Nothing we wear or apply to our skin can make us lose weight.

Yep, after all the years of research and inquiry, we now know what we knew before: there are few shortcuts to trimming off pounds. Serious weight loss requires serious pushing back from the table and moving that body more. That sounds about right.

UNDERSTANDING CARBOHYDRATES

Is it true, as some warn, that carbohydrates are the plague of our time? Or can we think more kindly of these energy-containing nutrients? If we could pose our questions to Mother Nature, this is what she might say:

What *are* carbohydrates? They are sugars and starches that occur in nature. Chemically, they are natural compounds made from the elements carbon, hydrogen and oxygen. Carbohydrates originate from the sun, the earth's source of energy. Plants receive that energy and convert it into the carbohydrate, glucose. This simple sugar fuels the production of more complex carbohydrates called starches. Much of the energy stored in fruit, grains, and vegetables is in the form of these carbohydrate molecules.

Are carbohydrates bad? You wouldn't be able to ask that question if they were! Most of the energy your body needs to think,

Quinn-Essential Nutrition

move, and work is in the form of one type of carbohydrate or another.

Can we lose weight if we cut carbohydrates out of our diets? You can lose weight if you cut anything that contains calories out of your diet; that includes carbohydrates, protein, fat and alcohol. Excess weight is simply an accumulation of stored calories from these sources.

Is it better to eat more protein and fewer carbs? That depends. We need valuable protein to keep our bodies in good repair and to arm our immune system. Brains also run on glucose; we need at least 130 grams of carbohydrates to fuel brain function each day.

Why do we lose weight so quickly when we cut the carbs?

Two possible reasons: It takes seven times as much water to convert protein, rather than carbohydrates, into energy. So when you severely restrict carbs, some of the weight you lose might be water. Another reason is that many of the foods we eat contain sugars and starches (carbohydrates). When we cut back on carbs, we aren't eating as much food or calories; and we lose weight.

Is it easier to burn fat on a low carbohydrate diet? Read your biology and physiology books. Without carbohydrates, our bodies cannot break down fat efficiently. A high intake of protein and fat without adequate carbohydrates forces the body to produce acids called ketones. If these substances build up too high in the blood, we should worry about our life, not our weight. Eating fewer than 100 grams of carbohydrates a day can put one at risk for an abnormal condition called "ketoacidosis."

Finally, consider this: When we unnecessarily restrict foods that contain carbohydrates, we also deny ourselves the nutritional benefits of whole grains, fruits and vegetables.

REFLECTION: Some popular books claim that carbohydrates are the brain's "silent killers" and the source of every evil on earth. Scientists who actually study such things however, conclude that diets rich in fruits and vegetables, whole grains, nuts and legumes (such as the well-studied DASH or Mediterranean diets) are associated with better cognitive, or brain function.

Archeologists estimate that mankind has been eating grains for at least the past 30,000 years. And I would guess that our ancestors didn't turn down fruit, berries or other carbs when they had the chance to eat. Glucose from these foods might have provided the energy they needed to run away from predators before they figured how to hunt them for food.

It's a fact that our brains run on glucose, a fuel derived from carbohydrates. Without glucose, brain cells die. Even on low carb diets, the body switches to other mechanisms to manufacture glucose for the brain; it's that important.

The World Health Organization (WHO) states that a higher intake of whole grains could helps alleviate early death and disability worldwide. And independent research by Consumer Reports states the "ideal diet is varied, rich in fruits and vegetables, whole grains, and low-fat dairy products plus modest amounts of fish and low-fat meat and chicken."

BEWARE THE HCG DIET

A favorite spoof on unproven nutrition products is an ad that states, "I lost $200 on bogus weight loss pills. Ask me how!" When it comes to weight loss methods, how do we know what to believe? Listen to trusted experts who don't jump at the chance to sell you something.

Dr. Mark Vierra is a respected bariatric (weight loss) surgeon at the Community Hospital of the Monterey Peninsula in California. Here are his comments on the hGC diet:

"Twenty years ago, patients used to report a diet history that included injections of the urine from pregnant mares. What a bizarre diet, I remember thinking. What I didn't know at the time was that they were describing the hCG diet."

In humans, a hormone called hGC (human chorionic gonadotrophin) is produced by the placenta when a woman becomes pregnant, Dr. Vierra explains. Its role is to stimulate the production of another hormone, progesterone, to maintain the lining of the uterus during pregnancy. The hGC hormone is a useful measure to determine if a woman is pregnant; and some fertility treatments use it to induce ovulation.

On the other hand, hGC is also produced in some rare forms of cancer. So how did it come to be used as a weight loss product?

"The hCG diet was first proposed by Dr. ATW Simeons in the 1950s," says Vierra. "He claimed that hCG could cause redistribution of fat and allow weight loss without hunger. He recommended a series of injections of the hormone in conjunction with a 500 calorie-a-day diet which was high in protein and low in carbohydrates."

The problem, says Vierra, is that it has clearly been shown that hCG has no effect on weight or fat distribution. Indeed, the US Food and Drug Administration (FDA) has concluded that over-the-counter HCG products marketed as weight loss aids are not only unproven, they are illegal.

"Many HCG products are marketed to be taken in connection with a very low calorie diet," Vierra adds. "It is the decrease in calories that accounts for any weight loss. There are currently no FDA-approved HCG products designed to help you lose weight."

Still, people who stick with the hCG diet lose weight. How? "Because a diet that calls for 500 calories per day and provides inadequate protein causes rapid breakdown of muscle rather than fat," says Vierra. "Starvation causes rapid weight loss, as does cancer, HIV, and other major infections or illness. Weight loss in this fashion is clearly unhealthy, causes rapid slowing of your metabolism, and is unhealthy in both the short- and long-term."

"No responsible scientist or physician has concluded that the hormone, hCG, can help you lose weight," says Vierra. His advice echoes that of the *American Society of Bariatric Physicians* that states in part, "The use of HCG for weight loss is not recommended."

If you want to get pregnant, hCG can be helpful, says Dr. Vierra. "But not if you want to lose weight in a healthy way."

Barbara A. Quinn, MS, RD, CDE

ARE YOU AN EASY KEEPER?

Our horseshoer commented that my friend's horse is a little plump. "What do you feed her?" he asked.

Just a small amount of hay in the morning and evening, she said.

"Oh," he said. "She's an easy keeper."

I learned that term long before I became a nutrition professional. When I was 12, I had a horse named Trinket. She was tall and lanky and barely had meat on her bones, except in summer when she snacked from the trees in our apple orchard.

My other horse, Sweetheart, was just the opposite. This full-figured mare got half the rations of her thin friend and still remained chubby. She was definitely an easy keeper.

What makes some of us Trinkets and others Sweethearts was the topic at a scientific session sponsored by the *American Diabetes Association*. If we are easy keepers, we may burn 200 to 300 fewer calories each day to do the same work as a person with a higher rate of metabolism, reported biomedical researcher Eric Ravussin, PhD. But we can improve our calorie-burning potential with regular physical activity.

New information has also emerged about how our bodies store fat. We used to think the human body could only manufacture new fat cells during certain stages of life, such as childhood and adolescence. And we assumed that weight gain after these stages of development were just making our existing fat cells bigger. Not true, said Swedish researcher Dr. Peter Arner. His studies show that humans continue to make new fat cells and those cells also continue to get bigger when we gain weight.

He also explained that our fat cells get smaller when we lose weight...but they don't go away. Unfulfilled, these fat-deprived adipose cells trigger the release of hormones that encourage us to eat more. This is one possible reason why people who lose weight often gain it back.

Is there any hope then, for us easy keepers? Yes, say experts, there is. Here are some recommendations:

- **Eat balanced meals at regular intervals.** Certain hormones in the digestive tract turn off the hunger switch when we have eaten a satisfying meal. And the best diet to stimulate the release of these hormones, says Dr. Stephen Bloom of the United Kingdom, is "a combination of protein, fat, and carbohydrates."
- **Fill up on high fiber foods.** Vegetables, whole fruit, and whole grain cereals and bread release non-digestible fibers into the lower gut that stimulate a hormone that turns off hunger.
- **Fidget.** People who can't sit still very long burn several hundred more calories a day than those who don't move much. Scientists call this "spontaneous physical activity."

I don't recall if my horse, Trinket, fidgeted more than Sweetheart. But they obviously had genetic differences. Trinket was programmed to be thin; Sweetheart's DNA clearly shouted "stout." Still, they munched the same type of diet, one high in plant fiber. Sweetheart just got smaller portions to maintain her filly figure. And they got regular meals and daily exercise to maintain their horsey vitality. Sounds like those are good habits for any easy keeper.

VITAMIN C AFFECTS WEIGHT

Long before I ever dreamed of becoming a registered dietitian, I saw my first case of nutritional deficiency. My pet guinea pig died of scurvy, a disease caused by a lack of vitamin C in the diet. I never saw his receding gums or heard him complain of joint pain which are common symptoms of this deficiency. I only recognized (too late) his lack of energy and vigor which can also signal low levels of vitamin C. It was only later that I learned vitamin C is an essential nutrient for guinea pigs as well as for humans.

Over the years, I personally have seen just one human case of scurvy, in an elderly man who lived alone and relied solely on canned and packaged foods. But that was a long time ago; everyone gets enough vitamin C these days, right?

Wrong, according to research by registered dietitian and vitamin C investigator Carol Johnson of Arizona State University. Her studies with supposedly healthy college students found more than a third had low levels of vitamin C in their blood. And this could be a big deal. Johnson's research suggests that even slight deficits on vitamin C intake may be one reason for our continual battle with obesity. Vitamin C affects how our body uses fat, she explains. In the body, it is used to make carnitine, a substance that helps our cells burn fat for energy. When vitamin C is in low supply, carnitine is lacking as well.

In her study, Johnson instructed one group of college "guinea pigs" to avoid vitamin C-rich foods such as oranges, grapefruit, strawberries, tomatoes, broccoli and sweet bell peppers. Another group supplemented their usual diet with 500 milligrams of vitamin C. In just two weeks, the students on low intakes of vitamin C had measurable decreases in their energy levels. And when they exercised, they burned less fat than the students with adequate levels of vitamin C.

Could it be, Johnson suggests, that a diet devoid of vitamin C-rich fruits and vegetables is a real nutritional reason for being too tired to exercise? Additionally, does a low intake of vitamin C interfere with our efforts to burn off fat? More studies are needed, she admits. But it's interesting, especially since her research found lower levels of vitamin C in the blood of people who were overweight.

How much vitamin C do we need? According to current guidelines, children need 15 to 65 milligrams (mg) of vitamin C a day. Adult women require 75 milligrams and men need 90 milligrams a day.

Here are some food sources: 1 red or yellow bell pepper (340 mg), 1 cup cooked broccoli (120 mg) 1 cup cooked Brussels sprouts (100 mg), 1 cup strawberries (80 mg), 1 orange (70 mg). More than adequate amounts of vitamin C exist in these foods. We just need to eat them.

REFLECTION: Further studies have confirmed that vitamin C plays an important role in the body's ability to synthesize carnitine, a molecule that burns fat for energy. In a 2006 study, Dr. Johnson and colleagues found that participants with a lower intake of vitamin C (40 milligrams a day) burned less fat during exercise than participants with higher intakes of vitamin C (400 milligrams a day).

YOU CAN BE TOO THIN

Maybe you can't be too rich but you can certainly be too thin. Serious health consequences result from being critically underweight. What is *too* thin? Think of it as the difference between leanness and gauntness. Athletes who are typically very lean have a high percentage of muscle mass and minimum stores of body fat. But even top athletes carry some essential body fat. Women need at least 12 percent of their body weight to be composed of fat and men need at least 3 percent to cushion our organs and to transport important fat-soluble vitamins such as vitamin D.

Granted, some of us have more than our fair share of body fat and may not really care to know for what higher purpose we were so endowed. By nature, women have more body fat than men; these extra stores of energy are required for bearing and feeding children. And it's these strategically placed fat stores that makes women softer and more rounded than our male counterparts.

One of the scariest eating disorders in the pursuit of thinness is anorexia nervosa, a life-threatening illness which results from an abnormal fear of becoming fat. Anorexia is characterized by these symptoms, according to the *American Psychiatric Association:*

1. An intense fear of gaining weight or becoming fat in spite of being obviously underweight;
2. Excessive dieting that leads to severe weight loss of 15 percent below one's expected weight for age, sex, and height. For example, a woman who is 5 feet 5 inches tall and normally weighs 125 pounds restricts her eating to drop her weight to 106 pounds;
3. Disturbed body image. A person with anorexia "feels" fat even when she is obviously emaciated.

What happens when the body becomes too thin? Self-imposed or not, the effects of starvation are very predictable. When deprived of life-sustaining nutrients and fuel, the body depletes all immediate sources of energy from muscle and fat cells; then it goes into survival mode.

Not knowing when or if the self-induced famine will end, the body begins to ration its few calories. Similar to turning a thermostat down to conserve fuel, the body begins to ration energy for basic body functions. In cases of extreme caloric restriction, a person's metabolism may drop by as much as 40 percent, say experts.

Body fat can be burned for energy but it cannot be turned into protein, an essential component of body organs and the immune system.

When denied adequate protein in the diet, the body is forced to break down its own protein stores from muscle and other vital tissue, including the heart. Ironically, when a person with anorexia loses the fat she fears, she also gives up the lean muscle she needs.

As anorexia progresses, vital body functions begin to turn off as the body desperately attempts to preserve itself; the heart beats slower, body temperature declines, and food is slowly or incompletely digested. Young females with this disorder may even stop having menstrual periods. Even with the body's valiant attempts to survive, the long-term result of self-imposed starvation is serious illness or death.

What is the treatment? Although nutrition therapy is crucial to restore the body to normal function, anorexia is primarily a psychological disorder. Thus, the primary goal of therapy is to help the patient conquer his or her fear of food and to understand and trust what it means to eat normally.

REFLECTION: According to the American College of Sports Medicine, a range of 10 to 22% body fat is considered healthful for men. And 20 to 32% is healthful for women. Body fat less than 3% for men and 12% for women is not adequate for the body's essential needs.

WILL'S WEIGHT LOSS PLAN

Will's doctor wants him to lose ten pounds before his knee surgery this summer; and he has asked me to help. "Just cut back on his food," Doc advises. I am therefore charged to make this as easy and non-threatening as possible. Right.

It's a familiar story: Will leads an active life; he is an athlete. He's never had a weight problem because he spends much of his time running all over creation. Even with a healthy appetite, he has never been overweight.

Then he hurt his knee. Now it hurts when he tries to run, so he sits and rests more. And he has gained weight which puts extra strain on his joints.

I am the dietitian, so of course, I want to help. I am aware that Will eats a well-balanced diet and most foods he eats with gusto. But now that his exercise is limited, he's eating too much. So I help him maintain a normal routine—same food, but in measured amounts. No longer does he get brimming bowls for dinner or the chance to nibble between meals.

I had hoped he wouldn't notice, that a little cut in quantity at each meal would be just fine with him. But he did notice; and it's hard to watch. As soon as he finishes breakfast, Will looks at me and his eyes say, "Is that all?" In the evening, he gobbles down dinner and when his pleadings for more are not effective, he retreats to bed. I try to explain that this is for his own good... that he will feel so much better when he loses weight and has less pressure on his injured joint. But it does not feel better to Will right now; and at times, he looks downright sad.

As the days go by, I begin to notice him less focused on food and more interested in other things of life, such as keeping an eye on the horses and digging up the garden. He is perkier and seems to be able to move around easier. And that makes us both happy. Yesterday, he didn't gobble down his breakfast. In fact, he actually left some in his bowl. And he wagged his tail to let me know he still loves me.

Surgery will hopefully resolve Will's incapacity. And in time, he will be running all over creation like Border collies do. And one day, he may realize that this was all indeed, worth it.

REFLECTION: My sweet Will lived a full and active life, running by my side through the hills of Garland Park in Carmel Valley for more than ten years. I still miss him.

NO MIRACLE IN MIRACLE DIET

So I'm killing time waiting for folks to show up for my supermarket tour. (Yes, I really do this.) And my eyes are drawn to an intriguing-looking product at the end of one aisle.

"Hollywood 48-hour Miracle Diet," the label boldly announces. "Lose up to 10 pounds in 48 hours!"

10 pounds in 48 hours? I wonder how it can do all that for only $14.99. I look closer at the label which instructs the buyer to mix 4 ounces of Miracle Diet into 4 ounces of water and sip on it for four hours. Repeat this three more times throughout the day. On Day 2, repeat the process.

Sounds simple enough; so what is in this formula that works such magic? Here are the ingredients, which are listed from the highest to the lowest amount by weight: Water, apple juice, orange juice, pureed apricot, peach, and banana, B-vitamins, and vitamins A, C, D, and E.

So this product is mostly water with fruit juice and nutrients commonly found in a multivitamin. What's the miracle?

I read a bit further. From the *Nutrient Facts* label, I calculate that this is an extremely low calorie diet, providing about 400 calories a day if I follow the instructions. I need about 1500 calories a day to fuel my basic body machinery. If I consume just 400 calories, it makes sense that my body would then dip into my fat stores for the other 1100 calories, right?

But wait. If every pound of body fat represents 3500 calories, I would need to burn off 35,000 calories in two days to lose "10 pounds in 48 hours." It is virtually impossible to burn off that much fat in that time period without a blow torch.

And herein lies another problem. Quick weight loss solutions don't just burn off excess body fat; they can starve the body of protein and cause it to burn up muscle. When this lean tissue is used for energy, water is lost. And even if it feels good when we step on the scale, it doesn't bode well for long-term strength or endurance. How much protein does this miracle product contain? Zero.

So let's be honest. If I feel like spending $14.99 on a mixture of vitamin-fortified fruit juice for a couple of days, this self-induced fast won't kill me. But can it really chip off 10 pounds in two days? I wouldn't bet on it. I keep reading and there it is...the disclaimer: "Weight loss based on fasting and moderate exercise. Individual results may vary." I'm sure they may.

Barbara A. Quinn, MS, RD, CDE

100-CALORIE DIFFERENCE

Obesity and type 2 diabetes go hand in hand, we learned at this meeting of diabetes educators in Washington, D. C. Sadly, both conditions have reached epidemic proportions and are driving health care costs through the roof. What's to blame? Not our genetics, experts told us. "There is nothing wrong with the human body," explained researcher Dr. John Peters. "It reacts exactly as it is supposed to in the environment it is placed."

For example, when we eat mostly high-fat, high-calorie foods and fight for a parking space close to the elevator that delivers us to our computers, our bodies most likely will gain weight. What is interesting, said Peters, is that the collective weight gain in this country over the past several years can be explained by just 100 extra calories a day. Over time, those extra calories accumulate to form excess body fat which, in some cases, can progress to type 2 diabetes.

On the positive side, we can effectively control our weight if we choose ways to eliminate 100 calories from our life each day by eating a bit less or moving a bit more. Aside from joining an Amish community where physical activity is a way of life and obesity and diabetes rates are low, Peters suggests we eliminate 100 "not needed" calories from our daily routines. Here are some ideas:

- Go an extra mile. Slap a pedometer on your belt and add 2000 more steps (about one mile) to your usual walking routine; this will burn off an extra 100 calories. Most experts recommend we work up to 10,000 steps a day (about five miles) if we are in good health.
- Order your latte or cappuccino with skim milk instead of whole milk; that will knock off 100 calories.
- Eat one less bite or portion of a high-calorie food each day. Each of these, for example, contains about 100 calories: one ounce of cheese; a tablespoon of cream, butter, oil or margarine; ½ cup of soda or other sweetened beverage; one ounce of rum, vodka, whiskey or other alcohol; five

ounces of wine, or two tablespoons of pancake syrup or salad dressing.
- Choose fruits and vegetables in place of higher calorie foods. One cup of cauliflower contains about 25 calories while the same amount of pasta or rice has close to 250 calories. It all adds up.

Melissa, a beautiful young lady, is a good example of this concept. "I didn't like vegetables until I was 20," she said as I watched her gobble down a plate of greens. "And I was getting pretty chubby, so I decided to start eating more fruit and vegetables to help me lose weight. And now I really like them!"

Over time, our bodies respond well to those 100-calorie deficits. It's a formula that works.

REFLECTION: Once we lose the weight, how do we keep it off? According to the National Weight Control Registry (NWCR), the largest prospective investigation of people who have lost 30 to 300 pounds and kept it off for more than five years, these daily habits are most important to long term weight management:
- *Continue to make reasonable choices about what and how much you eat;*
- *Exercise about one hour each day;*
- *Eat breakfast;*
- *Weigh yourself once a week and make adjustments to stay within your target weight range.*

AVOID WEIGHT ISSUES WITH KIDS

Dear Mom,

I've been thinking about you this week. I'm a nutrition professional, you know; and I am painfully aware of the difficulties faced by families with overweight children. At a nutrition symposium on this subject, respected weight management researcher James O. Hill told our group of nutrition experts that, back in the 1960's and 70's, obesity was not a problem in this country. What changed?

It's not just one thing, he said. "A lot of little things, over time, have added up to one big problem."

His comments took me back to my childhood. I was a chubby baby. I remember browsing through my baby photos and asking why you let me get so fat?

"You were always hungry," you said. Still, you and Dad did it right. You accepted each of your children as we were. My sister, Cheryl, was a skinny beanpole; Lynda and I were a bit more fluffy. You didn't try to change that.

I see that we were blessed back then. Outdoor play was the norm. You almost had to drag us into the house for dinner, especially in summer when we played endless hopscotch in the driveway or hide-and-seek with other kids in the neighborhood.

You gave us opportunities to be active each day. We had chores and regular house-cleaning duties to do. And you enforced Dad's rule that we could ride our horses as soon as we finished our tasks.

You made breakfast our usual routine. Interestingly, says Hill, people who eat a morning meal tend to consume 100 fewer calories by the end of each day than those who do not partake in a morning meal.

Granted, we didn't always choose a perfect diet. When I was a teenager, my friend Terry and I could eat most of the dough we had mixed for chocolate chip cookies before we ever got it baked. But I also recall that treats were few and far between. When we were young, you and Dad would pile us into the station wagon on Saturday nights and head for the drive-in movie with popcorn and sodas you packed from home. That was a special occasion.

We grew up knowing when to come to the table for breakfast and lunch and dinner. You established those times. And I remember our lively conversations around those meals. "Families that communicate are the key to good eating habits," says Hill. And a big part of that is family mealtime, he stressed.

Quinn-Essential Nutrition

During my teen years, I fretted about my weight and did not understand why I was not as slim as my friends. You and Dad were wise with that, too. You never nagged me about my weigh, whether it was up or down; and you consistently loved me.

I remember watching you eat slowly; and I marveled that you could leave food on your plate when you were no longer hungry. You modeled the smart habit of eating just until you felt satisfied, not full or stuffed. Research now confirms this strategy is a key to lifelong weight management.

Because of your example, Mom, I grew up with a strong memory of how meals are supposed to look. Yours were not fancy but, along with chicken, fish or meat and some type of starch like potatoes or rice, you *always* included a vegetable or two.

I remember when I came home for a visit after my first semester of college nutrition classes. You didn't bat an eye when I pointed out the obvious nutrient losses from your cooking methods. Your face lit up with a calm smile and you said, "I'm so thankful we managed to survive all these years before you went to college." You always said it just right.

REFLECTION: In 2013, a study reported in the Journal of the Academy of Nutrition and Dietetics confirmed that adolescents who eat breakfast and dinner meals with their family tended to have better quality diets than those who did not share these meals. And teens who ate breakfast with their families were less likely to be overweight.

A recent position paper by the Academy of Nutrition and Dietetics reports these effective strategies to help prevent and treat overweight children:

Start young. *Encourage healthful eating habits and physical activity in preschool-aged kiddos; this is a key time to help them maintain those habits as they grow.*

Promote water and milk as primary beverages *instead of juice and sugar-sweetened drinks. This strategy is strongly effective to lower the risk for young children to be overweight.*

Let kids practice good habits. *At school and home, give children opportunities to do fun physical activities and to eat tasty healthful foods.*

Focus on the positive. *Overweight kids do better over the long term when encouraged to choose more healthful foods instead of being told what not to eat, say experts.*

Protect growth. *Children are not little adults. Severe diets and food restrictions can seriously hamper a child's development.*

DIABETES DEFENSE

STEPS TO PREVENT DIABETES

I got a call from a family member...from his wife actually. Seems that hubby's doctor was concerned with the results from his recent blood tests. "He told us he has pre-diabetes, she said. "Should we worry?"

Maybe. His lab results did confirm the diagnosis of pre-diabetes, which is a fasting blood glucose between 100 and 125 or an A1C test between 5.7 to 6.4. According to the US Centers for Disease Control, up to half the people with pre-diabetes will develop type 2 diabetes within five years.

So how do we stop pre-diabetes from turning into full-blown type 2 diabetes? The answer comes from a landmark clinical trial in 2002 called the *Diabetes Prevention Program (DPP)*. In this study, people with pre-diabetes who took a medication called metformin reduced their risk for developing diabetes by 31 percent. But hold the presses; those who made changes in their lifestyle reduced their risk by 58 percent. And participants over the age of 60 who made these lifestyle changes lessened their risk for developing diabetes by a whopping 71 percent.

These are the lifestyle changes that helped prevent diabetes in this study:

1. **Lose some weight if you are overweight.** Participants who lost a modest 5 to 10 percent of their initial weight significantly lowered their risk.

2. **Cut the extra fat from your diet.** Diabetes risk went down when these people ate no more than a third of their daily calories from fat.
3. **Especially cut out saturated fat.** Why? Excess saturated fat contributes to insulin resistance which can lead to diabetes.
4. **Eat 25 to 35 grams of fiber each day.** In other words, a high fiber diet rich in fruit, vegetables, legumes, grains and other plant foods helped to prevent type 2 diabetes.
5. **Exercise at least 150 minutes every week.** Moving muscles use up glucose from the blood and improve the action of insulin. In this regard, physical activity works like a potent anti-diabetes medication. Because they benefit blood sugar levels and the body's use of insulin, exercise and weight loss are extremely effective in treating pre-diabetes, says Monterey, California endocrinologist, Dr. James Chu.

REFLECTION: According to the latest statistics by the US Centers for Disease Control and Prevention (CDC), more than a third (37 percent) of our population over the age of 20 now has pre-diabetes; more than half of those over age 65 are afflicted. This has led to the recent launch of the CDC's National Diabetes Prevention Program (DPP), a program that uses these proven strategies to reduce the risk for developing diabetes.

DIABETES QUIZ FOR LIFE

Dear Tom,

I hear your wife is nagging you about your diabetes. She doesn't think you take it seriously. And you don't like it when she withholds dessert and checks your breath for chocolate when you come home from work.

Quinn-Essential Nutrition

You know she just wants the best for you. And she wants you to avoid the complications that often come with uncontrolled diabetes—heart disease, kidney failure, blindness and amputations. But it doesn't have to be that way; most of the health problems linked to diabetes can be prevented by the choices you make…and not just about sugar. See how well you do on this quiz, adapted from information from the *American Diabetes Association* (www.diabetes.org):

1. If you have diabetes, the ABC's you need to know are: a) Avoid Bad Carbohydrates; b) A1c, Blood pressure, Cholesterol; c) Always Be Cautious. Answer: b.
2. A1C is a blood test that indicates your average blood sugar level over the past two to three a) months; b) days; c) Thanksgivings. Answer: a
3. If your A1C is higher than 7.0, you need: a) less dressing and gravy; b) more exercise; c) new medicine; d) a swift kick in the pants; e) a visit with your doctor and diabetes educator. Answer: e.
4. If you have diabetes, your blood pressure should be a) less than 130/80; b) checked often; c) controlled with diet, exercise and medications, if needed. All are correct.
5. DASH stands for a) Dietary Approaches to Stop Hypertension; b) Do Avoid Sodium Hikes; c) Don't Always Salt Ham. Answer: a
6. The DASH eating plan features blood pressure-regulating nutrients from a) fruits and vegetables; b) low fat dairy foods; c) nuts, beans and legumes; d) all of these. Answer: d.
7. Big meals can cause a surge of blood sugar (glucose) into your blood that a) makes your wife mad at you; b) creates "oxidative stress" that damages blood vessels and arteries; c) worsens your diabetes. Answers: b,c.
8. Carbohydrates are a) the devil; b) sugars and starches in foods; c) necessary for good health; d) found in fruit, vegetables, grains, beans, milk and yogurt. Answers: b,c,d

9. If you have diabetes, you can a) kiss pumpkin pie goodbye; b) eat moderate amounts of carbohydrates at each meal; c) eat candy when no one is looking; d) check your blood sugars two hours after a meal. Answers: b, d
10. In terms of carbohydrates, one cup of cooked rice or pasta can be expected to raise your blood sugar level as much as a) 3 slices of bread; b) 4 kiwi fruits; c) a partridge in a pear tree. Answers: a, b
11. Regular exercise a) lowers blood pressure, glucose and cholesterol levels; b) helps your body use insulin more efficiently; c) lets you leap over tall buildings in a single bound. Answers: a, b
12. If you are overweight, you can greatly improve your diabetes if you lose a) every bit of fat on your body; b) 7 to 10 percent of your current weight; c) your scale. Answer: b.

SLEEP AND DIABETES: WHAT'S THE CONNECTION?

We had not done this before. Two of us—one from our hospital's sleep center and the other from our diabetes program—sat listening intently to a teleconference on sleep apnea and diabetes. What does one have to do with the other? More than we previously realized, according to research findings from both fields.

Obstructive sleep apnea, or OSA, is characterized by disruptions in sleep caused by disordered breathing, explained sleep medicine physician Dr. Angela Hospenthal from the University of Texas Science Center. Symptoms of OSA include "heroic snoring" (the kind that can be heard through closed doors), waking up choking or gasping or with a dry mouth or sore throat, and being excessively tired during the day.

How do you know you have sleep apnea? Spend a cozy night in a sleep lab, hooked up to electrodes that measure how you breathe. Lots of physiological changes happen while sleep disordered folks snore, says Hospenthal. Oxygen and blood flow are reduced, blood pressure rises, and the heart experiences irregularities. It's not a restful sleep.

During waking hours, people with sleep apnea have trouble concentrating and remembering things, to which my sleep center expert nodded knowingly. And what does all this have to do with diabetes? Sleep apnea is linked to diabetes in several ways, we were informed.

Central obesity, excess weight we carry around the middle, puts us at risk for both sleep apnea and diabetes. "Fat cells in the upper body (apple shapes) have different health effects than fat cells in the hips and thighs," Hospenthal said.

Insulin resistance syndrome, a condition that often leads to diabetes, is also common in people with OSA. Why? When we don't breathe deeply, hormones are released that raise blood sugar levels and impair the body's ability to process blood sugar. We looked at each other and took a deep breath.

Neuropathy, nerve damage common in people with diabetes, is also prevalent in people with obstructive sleep apnea. No one knows exactly why.

So sleep apnea may lead to diabetes; and diabetes may lead to sleep apnea. And interestingly, when either condition is treated, the other tends to improve. For example, one effective therapy for sleep apnea is continuous positive airway pressure, or CPAP. And as this treatment helps get more oxygen to the body, it also helps control blood sugar levels. Here are other effective treatments for sleep problems and diabetes:

Lose excess weight. Even a modest weight loss (10 to 15 percent) decrease sleep problems and the risk for diabetes.

Avoid sleeping on your back. This position blocks airflow which can aggravate sleep problems and disrupt the body's ability to process blood sugar effectively.

Go to bed! Sleep deprivation is bad for your heart, your mind, and your body. Most adults require 6 to 8 hours of sleep each night. And avoid alcohol or other substances that can disrupt your sleep.

Barbara A. Quinn, MS, RD, CDE

AN IRISHMAN TALKS DIABETES

I sent an email to my new friend in the land of St. Patrick: "Top of the mornin' to you, Tom! Do they really say that in Ireland?"

He replied that the traditional greeting would be, "Hello Barbara." Then he added, "But there is some slang in different areas (of Ireland): 'Whatss aabout yee?' 'Augh am doing alright.' 'Cud be worse.'"

I met this cheerful Irishman while he was visiting his daughter, Avril and her husband, Jim in California. I fondly remember our first meeting. He strode over to the table where I was sitting and with a wide grin, said, "I'm Toum."

Toum? I repeated. Oh....Tom! Avril's dad! I shook his hand and we both smiled.

Tom told me he had recently been diagnosed with type 2 diabetes. And he admitted he was a bit confused about how to handle it. "When I went to the dietitian (in Ireland), she was a wee girl in her twenties. She kept asking me what I was eating and no matter what I said, she said, 'That's great!' and sent me off with a bit of paper."

I told him I would be happy to discuss his diet with him during his visit here. The following week, Avril invited me to have soup and a cup of tea with her dad. While we ate, Tom recounted his diagnosis and the instruction he had received from his vigilant daughter.

"I was eleven and half stone," he said.

I stared at him blankly until Avril interjected, "A stone is 14 pounds," she explained. We did the math.

"And when I got home from America, I was a waif," Tom continued. "I had lost a stone; I had to tell the girls in the chemist's shop who I was."

Chemist's shop? I repeated.

"The pharmacy," Avril said.

I asked Tom to tell me what he usually eats for breakfast.

"A plate of porridge..."

"Oatmeal," Avril interpreted.

"And sometimes bacon and eggs. We use potatoes a lot...and white bread."

Did he check his blood sugar values with a glucose meter? I asked. He produced a familiar machine, but the numbers were different from readings on American meters. I was a "wee" confused, until we realized that in Ireland, blood glucose is measured in millimoles per liter instead of milligrams per deciliter. When we did the conversion, I was happy to see that Tom's values were within normal ranges.

After lunch, Avril served up bowls of fresh strawberries with a "bit of cream." Do you eat desserts? I asked Tom.

"No, I don't eat sweets," he said.

His daughter looked at him sternly. "What about the apple tart?"

"Oh, yes, the apple tart...I thought you meant 'candies,'" he said with a grin. This initiated a conversation about carbohydrates, and a reminder that *all* forms of sugars and starches, from apple tarts to candies, affect blood glucose values.

Tom is back home in Ireland now. I recently emailed him to check on his progress. "Keeping to reasonable low (blood glucose) readings," he wrote. "Out on bicycle for 7 miles. Walked 4 miles on Monday and cut my helpings."

I asked him to describe his diet now that he's back home. "We have generally simple food; but then we have the Ulster fry, soda bread, potato bread, tomatoes, and black pudding."

Traditionally, he explained, if you visited older people unexpectedly, and they were out of fresh bread, they would say, "We have no bread; wud you take a bit of loaf?" I dare not ask about Ulster fry...

HELP KIDS DODGE DIABETES

Back in my rodeo days, a popular western song began, "Mommas, don't let your babies grow up to be cowboys. Don't let 'em pick guitar and drive them old trucks. Let 'em be doctors and lawyers and such." Times have changed. Today the song might be, "Mommas, don't let your babies grow up to be couch-boys. Don't let 'em text cell phones and sit on their tufts. Let 'em be active and playful and such."

Why the need to change our tune? We are in the midst of a global epidemic of type 2 diabetes in children, a phenomenom that did not even exist 20 or 30 years ago, says diabetes expert Francine Kaufman, MD. In the old days, a child diagnosed with diabetes most often had type 1, an autoimmune disorder that destroys the body's ability to make the hormone, insulin. Type 2 diabetes—a condition related to aging, obesity and inactivity—was rarely seen in children.

As our children have become heavier and more sedentary, the diagnosis of type 2 diabetes is more common. Family history plays a role, too, says Kaufman. Moms and dads can pass on a genetic propensity for type 2 diabetes to their children. But they can also take steps to prevent this disease in their kiddos. Here are some ideas:

Momma's, don't let your pregnancies be complicated by excessive weight gain. Too much weight packed on during pregnancy increases a child's risk for developing type 2 diabetes later in life.

Let 'em be breastfed until at least 6 months of age. Besides getting top-notch nutrition, breastfed babies are less likely to be obese or to develop type 1 or type 2 diabetes, says Kaufman.

Daddies, do all you can to keep your kids active. Physical movement helps a child maintain a normal weight; and active play is a powerful "medicine" against type 2 diabetes, say experts.

Don't let them gulp sodas and sugary drinks. Little bodies respond to big doses of liquid sugar with a robust insulin response, says Kaufman. Over time, this puts a strain on the pancreas, the organ that makes insulin. "No drinking sugar, including juice," is Kaufman's advice for most children. Give toddlers only small amounts of juice and dilute with water.

Let 'em eat salads and whole grains and fruit. Because the stirrings of type 2 diabetes can start in the womb, it can hit much more aggressively in children than in adults. Start early with reasonable eating and exercise habits to keep little cowpokes from becoming too heavy; kids who dodge obesity are likely to dodge type 2 diabetes as well.

"Prevention should be the focus," says Kaufman. Amen to that, cowboys and cowgirls!

UNDERSTANDING THE GLYCEMIC INDEX

"What's the glycemic index of avocados?" a co-worker asked as she munched on a piece of cheese wrapped in a lettuce leaf. "The diet book I'm reading does not have it on the list." I looked up from my computer and gave her the simple answer. Avocados are high in fat; they contain few if any carbohydrates, the sugars and starches that affect the glycemic index (GI) of foods.

What is the Glycemic Index? "It's not a simple measure," said Katherine Beals, associate professor at the University of Utah who spoke on this topic at a meeting of the California Dietetic Association. "The accurate definition of glycemic index is very complex because the concept is complex."

I'll say. Glycemic Index was first developed in 1987 by researchers at the University of Toronto to compare how a specific weight (50 grams) of different foods affects the uptake of glucose (sugar) into the bloodstream of various individuals. These responses were measured for two hours after eating each food and were compared to how this individual responded to a "reference food" such as white bread. Stay with me here...The difference between the rise in a person's blood sugar for the test food compared to the reference food became known as the "glycemic index" or GI. Whew.

In general, foods with a higher GI produce a higher peak in blood sugars within 2 hours of eating than do foods with a lower GI. Who cares? People with diabetes do; this condition can cause blood sugars to skyrocket after meals. Unfortunately, said Beals, the Glycemic Index is not as simple as some would hope. Here are some facts:

- Different individuals respond differently to different foods. A person with diabetes, for example, will have a different blood glucose rise after drinking a glass of orange juice than will a marathon runner.
- Over time, the same person can respond differently to the same food. A bagel, for instance, might make your blood sugar jump high one day and stay normal the next time. How we respond to carbohydrate foods is highly variable, said Beals.
- The GI of a specific food varies widely. Early reports targeted carrots as high glycemic index, for example. Recent and more reliable research gives carrots a low GI.
- Quantity matters. The Glycemic Index of a food is based on a fixed weight (50 grams or approximately 2 ounces) of that food. If you eat more or less of that amount, the GI gets a bit fuzzy.
- Maturity matters. Ripe bananas have a higher GI than green bananas, for example.
- Preparation method matters. How a food is chopped, mashed, cooked or processed affects its glycemic index. One easy way to lower the GI of your diet, Beals joked, is to "swallow your food whole."
- Low GI does not always translate to the healthiest foods. Hot dogs without the bun and beer have a lower GI than vegetarian pizza. And this begs the question, What's our real goal here? Using the GI as the end-all to eating, says Beals, sends mixed and often wrong messages. Her advice? Use the Glycemic Index as one guide, not the only one, to understand how food affects your blood sugar levels, especially if you have diabetes. Choose a healthy variety of foods in your diet, including carbohydrates. It doesn't need to be complicated.

WINNING THE GOLD AGAINST TYPE 1 DIABETES

He's an Olympic hero. Swimmer Gary Hall won ten Olympic medals—five gold, three silver, and two bronze. And what makes his career extra-amazing is that Hall has type 1 diabetes, a condition that prevents his body from making insulin, a vital hormone that transfers energy (glucose) into the cells of his body. He therefore must inject insulin into his body several times a day to survive.

"When I was first diagnosed in 1999," says Hall, "I was told I wouldn't be able to continue my swimming career at the level I was used to competing. Then I was referred to a great endocrinologist and a crack team of specialists—a diabetes nurse educator, dietitian, and exercise physiologist. These medical professionals put together a program that enabled me to control my diabetes and get back into training."

Hall went on to win medals in the 2000 and 2004 Summer Olympic Games, including consecutive gold medals in the 50-meter freestyle. He provided these insights about type 1 diabetes and high level competition:

"Leading up to the Olympics, it was almost eight hours of training, six days a week. When you are exercising that much, your body needs carbohydrates (sugars and starches from fruit, vegetables, bread, cereals, pasta, milk and yogurt) for fuel. I test my blood sugar 5 to 8 times every day. On competition days, it could be as many as 16 times through the day...at least once an hour."

Why so often? "There are days when you can do everything you are supposed to do and there's going to be fluctuations in your blood glucose levels that you just can't explain. For example, the different types of exercise we do affects how much insulin is required. Aerobic training would drop my blood sugars as much as a couple hundred points within 40 minutes. Then on days that we trained in the weight room or did short sprints in the pool, that didn't lower my blood glucose anywhere near as much. So you have to anticipate how your body will react."

Stress hormones can also wreak havoc on blood glucose levels, says Hall. "The pressure of competing in the Olympics…I can't even describe it. For example, my 50 meter freestyle usually took me 21-some seconds." (Easy for him to say.) "I would shoot for my blood glucose levels to be around 150 before the race. After a short race, they were in the high 300's. As soon as I got out of the pool, it was important for me to get insulin right away so I could eat carbohydrates to re-power and re-fuel my muscles."

It's a juggling act, Hall admits, to balance exercise with nutrition and insulin. "Even Olympic athletes can get burned out and discouraged. But we live in a time that diabetes is now manageable. So take advantage of it. It's powerful and true; you can do anything you want to do."

REFLECTION: Gary Hall, Jr., was inducted into the United States Olympic Hall of Fame in July, 2012.

RESEARCHING THE RESEARCH

NUTRITION ALTERS GENES

Genes and nutrition, both are critical for laying the foundation of our health; and both can modify the extent of our wellness, says registered dietitian Connie Hurlbert. Nutritional genomics, the study of how our genetic code is affected by components in food, had barely emerged into the scientific world in 2008 when she reported this from an international symposium at the University of California at Davis:

"It's in my genes," sounds positive when your friend smiles and explains how she can consume all the French fries off her plate (and yours) and her waistband doesn't budge. On the other hand, this same friend who wears size zero jeans may also tell you her cholesterol is never under 400. (Normal is less than 200.)

What we eat and how we are put together genetically influence the delicate balance between health and disease, according to a new field of research called "nutrigenomics." It began with the completion of the Human Genome project in 2003, according to the Center of Excellence in Nutritional Genomics (CENG) at the University of California at Davis. Now we want to understand how food affects our genes and how our genetic differences influence the ways we respond to nutrients in food.

Why do we respond differently to the different diets, for example? Or why can some people drink cow's milk without problems and others cannot? Our genetic makeup plays a role. Researchers have identified a genetic "variant" that is responsible for the ability to digest lactose, the sugar in milk. People who widely consume milk, such as Northern Europeans, are more apt to carry this particular genetic material than people of Southeast Asia, for instance. In fact, 95 percent of people from Northern European descent drink milk with no trouble. But only 2 percent of those genetically tied to Southeast Asia tolerate milk from cows.

Clearly, our genetic differences influence whether we get essential calcium from cow's milk or from other sources such as fortified soy milk. And it helps us see how one set of food recommendations may not be optimal for every individual.

Other topics being studied from the perspective of nutrigenomics include individual tolerances to caffeine and how the hormone leptin affects hunger and appetite in different people. And nutrigenomics may soon become a tool to prevent, delay and treat chronic diseases like obesity, cancer, and heart disease. In the near future, you may meet with a registered dietitian for an individualized diet based on your own unique genetic profile.

REFLECTION: Our current understanding of how our genetic profile might pre-dispose us to develop diseases like cancer and heart disease has undergone a major paradigm shift, say experts. Just as we have genes that determine the color of our eyes, we now know of genes that affect our susceptibility for disease. What is new and exciting from a nutrition perspective is that certain genes can be switched on or off by triggers in our environment. Animal studies, for example, have shown that a high-fat diet in pregnancy can change the expression of genes in the offspring which sets them up to be overweight or to develop type 2 diabetes. Words like "epigenic programming" and "imprinted genes" may one day better explain why different people respond to different foods in different ways.

Instead of individual foods, patterns of eating are emerging as the most powerful way to shift our genetic expression towards health. For example, a 2013 Canadian study found that diets with a high proportion of vegetables, fruits, and whole grains and low intakes of refined grains, sweets and processed meats may help turn off the activity of genes which promote cancer growth.

Certain nutrients such as choline, folic acid and other B-vitamins provide methyl groups involved in gene expression as well, say researchers. If these components are missing, our "good health-expressing" genes may not be activated. One more reason to make sure our daily diets are balanced in all essential nutrients.

Nutrition genomics is still in its infancy, but we still know what we already knew, say experts. The optimal diet to fuel our disease-fighting genes is one similar to the Mediterranean way of eating: rich in fruits, vegetables, whole grains, and fish and limited in highly refined grains, sweets and processed meats. Here are some of the compounds in this type of diet that can turn on genes to suppress cancer growth:

- *Sulforaphane and isothiocyanates: broccoli, kale, cabbage*
- *Organo-selenium compounds: garlic*
- *Biotin: chard, egg yolk*
- *Alpha-lipoic acid: green leafy vegetables such as spinach*

Questions will continue to emerge as we move forward with this science of nutrigenomics. According to a 2014 position paper on this topic by the Academy of Nutrition and Dietetics, legal and ethical issues will also need to be addressed.

COCONUT OIL UPDATE

I'm staring at a really cute picture of my granddaughter and I smile. I shuffle through other pictures on my computer and smile again at the coconut-covered bunny cake I made for Easter. And I wonder, based on what we know and don't know about coconut fat, if I should embrace my coconut friend…or not? Maybe neither, according to a variety of reputable sources. Here are some facts:

1. According to the Library of Congress, coconut is a fruit that covers a seed (like a peach or an olive), affectionately called a "drupe."
2. Most (almost 90 percent) of the oil derived from coconuts is the saturated variety, a type of fat that tends to raise blood cholesterol levels in humans.
3. About 46 percent of the saturated fat in coconut oil is lauric acid, a fat of "medium chain" length that raises beneficial HDL cholesterol as well as harmful LDL cholesterol levels in the blood. This is why some believe coconut oil may be good for heart health. But wait...
4. Another one-third (about 30 percent) of the fats in coconut oil are myristic and palmitic acids, considered to be detrimental saturated fats in terms of their affect on serum cholesterol levels.
5. A small percentage (about 3%) of the fat in coconut oil is stearic acid, a neutral saturated fat that tends to be neither good or bad for blood cholesterol levels. (By the way, about a third of the saturated fat in beef and cocoa butter is neutral stearic acid as well.)
6. Coconut oil also contains a small amount (about 9 percent) of healthful unsaturated fats (oleic and linoleic acid); these are also found in abundance in oils such as canola and olive oil.
7. Food labels clump all the saturated fat content of a food into one category, the healthful as well as the beneficial. And herein lies the confusion. For example, even "good fat" olive oil contains a small percentage of palmitic acid, a saturated fat that can be detrimental to blood cholesterol levels. And lean beef which is considered a source of "bad" fat actually contains a lower percentage of detrimental palmitic and myristic fatty acids than coconut oil.

8. Still, strong evidence shows that populations of people who eat a diet high in saturated fat have a higher rate of diseases of the heart. And in general, when saturated fat intake increases, so does bad LDL cholesterol.
9. As for coconut oil, experts from the University of California, Berkeley Wellness Center conclude: "You should limit these oils since their effects on cholesterol are not fully understood. You can use coconut oil in cooking on occasion if you like the flavor. Vegetable oils such as canola, olive, soy, or safflower are recommended for day-to-day use, however."

Alas, in terms of heart disease, coconut oil may not be the "miracle fat" some had hoped for. We need to remember that various mixtures of good and bad exist in all foods. That said, Mr. Bunny Cake is here to stay...but only for special occasions.

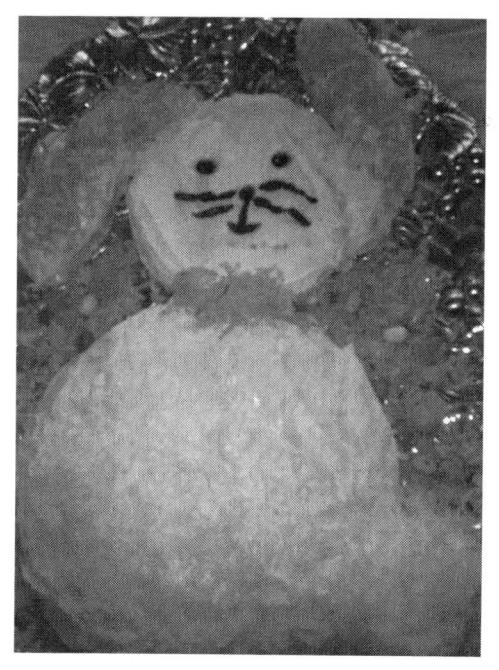

Mr. Bunny Cake

REFLECTION: Coconut oil and its effects on health continue to be studied and debated. Clinical evidence is still lacking on its reported benefit for heart health, however. According to Dariush Mozaffarian, MD, DrPH, of Harvard Medical School and Harvard School of Public Health, "We still don't know if it (coconut oil) is harmful or beneficial."

Dr. Walter Willett, also from Harvard School of Public Health, writes, "for now, I'd use coconut oil sparingly. Most of the research so far has consisted of short-term studies to examine its effect on cholesterol levels. We don't really know how coconut oil affects heart disease. And I don't think coconut oil is as healthful as vegetable oils like olive oil and soybean oil, which are mainly unsaturated fat and therefore both lower LDL and increase HDL. Coconut oil's special HDL-boosting effect may make it 'less bad' than the high saturated fat content would indicate, but it's still probably not the best choice among the many available oils to reduce the risk of heart disease."

ORGANIC JUNK FOOD

Organic jelly beans. Organic potato chips. Organic vodka. No matter what the product, the term "organic" is perceived as being healthier than other foods, said registered dietitian Sharon Palmer in an article in *Environmental Nutrition*.

So what does the term "organic" really mean? According to the United States Department of Agriculture (USDA) which regulates organic standards, organic food is produced without the use of most conventional pesticides, synthetic fertilizers, bioengineering, or ionizing radiation. In other words, it refers to how a food is farmed.

Organic does not necessarily mean a food can't be highly processed, however. Any food that has been changed in some way from its original form is considered processed. Take a chocolate chip cookie...OK, take two. Organic chocolate chip cookies are made with organically cultivated wheat, sugar, butter and chocolate. But the organic flour and sugar can still be refined and white. And the nutritional value of these cookies may be no different from regular cookies. Excess fat and calories from organic treats are no less damaging than those from other foods.

So while organic farming methods help ensure healthy soil and ecosystems, organic standards do not regulate a food product's nutritional attributes, says Palmer. A product made with organic brown rice syrup or evaporated cane juice still contains sugar. And if organic sweetened beverages, candy bars, and chips are stripped of healthful nutrients, they're just organic junk food.

What about organic milk? It comes from cows who were fed organic feed and were not given hormones or certain types of medications for illness. Both organic and regular milk contain the same profile of essential nutrients, say nutrition experts. And both types of milk are enriched with vitamin D, a hormone-like vitamin that helps the body absorb calcium. Thankfully, all milk, organic or not, is strictly tested for antibiotic or pesticide residues to ensure these are not present in milk.

One interesting note: Some organic milk may last longer than regular milk because of how it is processed, according to Craig Baumrucker, professor of animal nutrition and physiology at Pennsylvania State University. Because organic milk is not produced in all parts of the country, it may have to travel farther to reach stores. To help it stay fresh longer, it may be treated with UHT (Ultra High Temperature) which destroys most all its bacteria content. This method of destroying harmful bacteria imparts a slightly sweeter taste to organic milk, says Baumrucker. UHT is different from pasteurization, which kills most but not all bacteria. (That's why we need to refrigerate milk and drink it within a few days.)

Organic or not, health experts still call us to choose from whole grains, fresh fruit, vegetables, beans and legumes, low-fat dairy foods and lean meats, poultry and fish..and an occasional cookie.

Barbara A. Quinn, MS, RD, CDE

MILK THISTLE: WEED OR MEDICINE?

Funny what you find in your own backyard. Friends were helping me whack some pretty tall weeds when Pat, a horticultural expert, noticed one that did not look particularly friendly. "That's a milk thistle," he said, pointing to the plant I was attacking with my shovel. "I believe it's got some therapeutic value."

I commented how very interesting that was and kept whacking. But the next day, I dug into some references from the National Center for Complementary and Alternative Medicine (NCCAM). Sure enough, this spiny purple-flowered plant has a long history as a remedy for a variety of ailments. And according to *Rational Phytotherapy*, a classic science-based guide to herbal medicine, that ugly looking weed I chopped to the ground is considered one of the few plant-based medicines to have undergone well-controlled, pharmacologic testing.

Milk thistle, named for the whitish fluid in its leaves, is a prickly member of the daisy family. Its Latin name is *Silybum marianum;* and the fruit of this plant contains a group of active compounds collectively called "silymarin." Some studies have shown that this substance exerts a beneficial effect on the liver, helping to reduce inflammation and repair the cells of this vital organ. And while it is impossible to get volunteers for a study to see if milk thistle improves the survival rate after accidental mushroom poisoning, there are several published reports that people treated with milk thistle infusion after eating the deadly "death cap" mushroom had higher rates of survival.

To date, says the NCCAM, there is no conclusive evidence to prove all the claimed uses for milk thistle. However, several large research studies are in process to look at this herb's usefulness for cancer prevention and to treat hepatitis.

Stinging nettle, another not-so-nice-sounding plant that stings the skin like tiny hypodermic needles, has also been studied for its beneficial health effects. Some people even eat stinging nettle as a vegetable. Cooking apparently deactivates the chemical on its leaves responsible for its painful sting.

One of the most interesting cures for arthritis in centuries past was a good flogging with stinging nettle branches. The resulting pain and inflammation was reported to relieve the joint pain, or at least make the patient forget about it for a while. Recent clinical trials have found that an extract from the root of this plant provided some relief from an enlarged prostate. Other studies on animals found that stinging nettle preparations could lower blood pressure and blood glucose levels.

A word to the wise, cautions the NCCAM: The fact that many plants and herbs have active ingredients means these active ingredients can also interact with other substances. Stinging nettle is a source of vitamin K, for example, which could interact with anticoagulant (blood thinning) medicine.

Herbal products may also contain ingredients that increase or decrease the effectiveness of certain medications. Unfortunately, the strict rules that apply to the safety and effectiveness of prescription drugs do *not* apply to dietary supplements. And sometimes, what is implied on the label is not what is in the bottle. Always notify your physician if you take supplements or herbs for any reason...even if it springs from your own backyard.

REFLECTION: According to the National Cancer Institute at the National Institutes of Health (NIH), silymarin and silybin (the active ingredients in milk thistle) appear to protect the liver by blocking toxins from entering the cell or by moving toxins out of the cell before damage can occur. And while a few case reports and clinical studies show promise, the US Food and Drug AdminIstration (FDA) has not approved the use of milk thistle for the treatment of any medical condition.

Barbara A. Quinn, MS, RD, CDE

MAKE WHEY FOR DAIRY

Little Miss Muffet sat on her tuffet eating her curds and whey... which may have helped her shapely figure. Whey and other components in dairy foods are being studied for their effects on body weight, according to Dr. Michael Zemel, nutrition researcher from the University of Tennessee. "We know that a dairy-rich diet helps in weight loss in people who are counting calories, roughly doubling the effectiveness of calorie cutting alone. And that would be by incorporating three servings of milk, cheese or yogurt into the daily diet."

How can this be? Calcium has what Zemel calls an "anti-obesity effect." His studies found people on weight loss diets lost more weight and fat when they ate a high calcium diet (1200 milligrams calcium daily) compared to a low calcium diet (400 milligrams a day). (One cup of milk or yogurt contains approximately 300 milligrams of calcium.) Zemel's research also found that people who got their calcium from dairy foods lost more weight and fat than those who got their calcium from supplements or calcium-fortified foods.

"When you don't have enough calcium in your diet," he explains, "your body releases hormones to help your body retain calcium. One of those hormones, calcitriol, unfortunately also sends messages to your fat cells that interfere with the biochemical machinery involved with fat breakdown. When you get adequate calcium in your diet, you suppress that hormone, so your fat cells can more normally break down and burn fat."

Why do dairy foods have a greater effect on weight loss than calcium from other sources? That's what Zemel wanted to know. He began to look at other components in dairy foods. "Just like the nursery rhyme, we separated milk into curds (casein) and whey, two distinct proteins. The extra good stuff turns out to be in the whey."

The types of protein in whey help protect muscle during weight loss, says Zemel. Whey protein contains leucine, an essential amino acid used to synthesize muscle tissue. Studies have found that a diet high in leucine helps store protein into muscles.

Along came a spider...pardon me for being skeptical. "I was skeptical myself," says Zemel, who says his research on dairy and calcium has been corroborated by 50 other research papers outside his lab. "I did not publish this for 12 years...until we were able to understand the mechanism."

"Let's be clear, however," he adds. "It's not as simple as drinking three glasses of milk a day to lose weight. Calcium and dairy foods do not erase calories. Calories absolutely count."

Zemel also disclosed that a substantial portion of his research is funded by the dairy industry. "I make no bones about it, pardon the pun," he said. "Quite frankly, I will take money for my research from anyone who will give it to me as long as there are no strings attached. And that is the case with anyone's work with the Dairy Council. Not all the work in this field was supported by the dairy industry however. Many people who published corroborating data have done so from databases that were not industry funded"

And that did not frighten Miss Muffet away.

REFLECTION: While the evidence is still inconclusive, a study published in the December, 2013 issue of the Journal of the Academy of Nutrition and Dietetics reported that older women (70 to 85 years of age) who consumed about two cups of milk, yogurt or cheese each day had greater lean body mass and better physical performance than women of the same age who ate fewer dairy foods.

Researchers have yet to identify all the components in dairy foods that may explain these benefits. High quality protein, calcium and certain growth factors in dairy foods may enhance muscle mass, they theorize. And whey protein can help rebuild muscle mass following exercise, according to recent studies. Part of this effect may be due to the easy digestion and absorption of whey protein. Whey also contains a high amount of the amino acid, leucine, a protein building block that signals protein to accumulate in muscles.

Barbara A. Quinn, MS, RD, CDE

IS SUGAR ADDICTIVE?

Am I addicted to sugar? I asked myself after I polished off a piece of pumpkin pie with whipped cream. According to a recent article in *Food and Nutrition*, a publication of the *Academy of Nutrition and Dietetics*, yummy food stimulates the same pleasure centers in the brain that are stimulated by addictive drugs like cocaine. And just like drug abusers, I could become so "hooked" on tasty food that I seek it even when I know the consequences might be painful. Gulp.

Granted, most of the research on this topic has been conducted on animals, not humans. Researchers at Princeton University for example, found that rats prefer sugar water to plain water. And when the sweet stuff is taken away, they go through symptoms of withdrawal. Other rats studied at Scripps Research Institute ran away from their chow bowl when they heard a signal that warned them of an impending electrical shock. But the story changed when these rats were fed chocolate, cheesecake, and sausage. When they heard the signal, they kept eating...even when they knew pain was on the way.

Of course, humans are not rats...most of the time. And scientists have never observed true withdrawal symptoms by depriving humans of flavorful foods. So the jury is still out. But if food addiction really does exist, sugar may not be the lone culprit. It's probably a combination of sugar, fat, and salt that triggers addictive-type behavior in humans, say scientists. Toffee, anyone?

LOWDOWN ON SUGAR SUBSTITUTES

A reader asked, "I would like to know the difference between all the substitute sugars on the market. My son has diabetes. What can I use that won't affect his blood sugar and tastes like regular sugar?"

Perhaps the only sugar that truly "tastes like regular sugar" is sucrose, what we refer to as table sugar. It contains 16 calories and 5 grams of carbohydrates per teaspoon. People with diabetes can eat small amounts of regular sugar, if they understand how to match their carbohydrate intake (sugar is a carbohydrate) to their blood sugar goals.

"Non-nutritive" sweeteners are substitutes for sugar that contain minimal amounts of carbohydrates and calories; they therefore do not affect blood sugar levels. And bonus, they do not promote tooth decay like regular sugar. Here are some common sweeteners approved for use in the United States:

- Saccharin is the pink packet, or *Sweet and Low*. Warning labels hung over saccharin for many years after the US Food and Drug Administration (FDA) determined that large amounts of this sweetener pumped into mice increased their risk for bladder cancer. In 2000, after a thorough review of new findings, saccharin was officially removed from the list of potential carcinogens; and it has regained its status as a safe sweetener.
- Aspartame is the blue packet sweetener known as *Equal* or *NutraSweet*. One of the most intensely studied sweeteners, aspartame is approved for use in more than 100 countries. Contrary to what you might read on the internet, this substance does not turn to poison when it is heated to high temperatures; it just loses its sweetness. And concern that aspartame breaks down to methanol and cause vision loss? A glass of tomato juice contains six times more methanol than a beverage with aspartame, say food scientists. Although some people report allergic reactions to aspartame, at least two well-controlled double-blinded studies (people did not know if they were ingesting aspartame or not) failed to confirm these suspicions. Neither has this sweetener been found to be related to cancer or multiple sclerosis, as some have feared.

    Made from two protein building amino acids (aspartic acid and phenylalanine), aspartame carries a warning label for people with a rare genetic disorder called phenylketonuria or PKU. These individuals cannot digest phenylalanine and should therefore avoid aspartame.

- Sucralose (brand name *Splenda*) holds up well at high temperatures and many think it tastes closer to regular sugar than previous sweeteners. Sucralose is made from a molecule of sucrose (sugar) that is modified with chlorine atoms. Is that safe? More than 100 studies over the past 30 years have shown that it is. Since the body does not recognize sucralose as a real sugar, it does not break it down or absorb it. Therefore it passes through the body relatively unchanged.
- Nectresse™ is a no calorie sweetener made with Monk fruit, a green melon that grows on mountaintops in Asia. Sugar extracted from this fruit is 150 times sweeter than cane or beet sugar, so very little goes a long way. Nectresse also contains erythritol, a sugar alcohol produced by the fermentation of another type of sugar called dextrose. This sweetener is considered a "free" food for people with diabetes because it contains less than five grams of carbohydrate (sugar) per serving. Nectresse is heat stable and can therefore be used in cooking and baking. One-fourth teaspoon equals the sweetness of 1 teaspoon sugar.
- Stevia is an herb native to the highlands of South America and a member of the chrysanthemum family. Leaves from the stevia plant yield an extract that is 200 times sweeter than regular sugar. Some describe its taste as "licorice-like." In 2009, the US Food and Drug Administration approved rebaudioside A, an extract from stevia leaves, for use as a sweetener. This purified extract is "Generally Recognized as Safe" (GRAS) by the FDA. One product that contains this extract is called Truvia®.

REFLECTION: The use of sweeteners continues to be controversial. In 2013, the peer-reviewed Journal of Food and Chemical Toxicology reaffirmed the safety of aspartame as a sweetener. Looking at studies over the past two decades, these researchers found no association between aspartame use and cancer, cardiovascular disease, or other medical problems. Also in 2013, the European Food Safety Authority (EFSA), after undergoing "one of the most comprehensive risk assessments of aspartame ever undertaken," reaffirmed the safety of aspartame.

Some studies suggest that low-calorie sweeteners interfere with appetite regulation and might be responsible for our expanding waistlines. In 2014, an extensive review on this subject concluded that low-calorie sweeteners do not lead to food cravings or weight gain. Yet another 2014 study on mice and humans suggested that artificial sweeteners alter bacteria in the gut and change the body's ability to keep blood sugar levels normal. Stay tuned.

D-LATEST ON THE SUNSHINE VITAMIN

Vitamin D in tandem with calcium is extremely important to the health of our bones, a fact confirmed by more than 1000 research studies. However, the effects of this vitamin in other areas of health are less clear.

Even determining how much vitamin D we need is complicated. Our skin can synthesize it when exposed to sunlight. But unless we are regularly outdoors without sun screen, we will need to consume vitamin D from our diet or from supplements. According to the latest Dietary Guidelines for Americans, everyone from 1 to 70 years of age needs about 400 to 600 International Units (IU) of vitamin D a day. Older people require 800 IU's per day.

Certain groups of people are more at risk for vitamin D deficiency, say experts. Older people, those who live indoors most of the time, and dark-skinned individuals are most at risk. Supplemental vitamin D is highly recommended for these folks.

To protect us from getting toxic doses of vitamin D, the Institute of Medicine (IOM) has set Tolerable Upper Intake (UL) limits for vitamin D. These are the upper levels of intake, from food and supplements combined, which have not been shown to pose any adverse health effects. For children ages one to three years of age, for example, the UL for vitamin D is 2500 IU. It's 3000 IU for children four to eight years of age and 4000 IU for older children and adults. Best not to exceed these amounts unless directed by a medical professional. Vitamin D in doses higher than 10,000 IU per day could damage the kidneys and other body tissues, says the IOM. More is not always better.

What's a normal level of vitamin D that we should look for on a blood test? Most labs report a normal range of 25-hydroxy vitamin D (the typical blood test to determine vitamin D status) between 30.0 to 74.0 nanograms per milliliter (ng/mL). Our current Dietary Guidelines for Americans state that 20 ng/ml is adequate for most people.

REFLECTION: At the 2013 Linus Pauling Institute Diet and Optimum Health Conference, noted vitamin D researcher Robert Heaney of Creighton University reported that serum levels of vitamin D below 32 nanograms/milliter may trigger bone pain (osteomalacia) and poor absorption of calcium. Higher levels of vitamin D appear to assist in the body's response to insulin, the hormone that helps control blood glucose (sugar) levels. Based on this and other evidence, Heaney estimates our optimal blood levels of vitamin D are more in the 40 to 60 mg/mL range. Again, this blood test is commonly referred to as "25-OH vitamin D."

Other interesting findings on vitamin D: It is involved in the expression of about one of every ten genes in our genetic code. Adequate amounts of vitamin D have been found to help prevent breast cancer and heart disease. And a 2013 study on seniors 55 years and older found that a vitamin D deficit made it doubly difficult to walk up and down stairs and get in and out of a chair.

GRASS FED BEEF

From the beaches of California to the sand hills of Nebraska, my daughter, like her mom, has become an expert in nutrition. She just works with a different type of clientele. Stephanie is a ruminant nutritionist; her clients are real cows. On a recent visit to western Nebraska, we bumped around in a feed truck at the university research facility she helps to manage. Here I began to see the difference between her specialty and mine.

Ruminant animals have a rumen, the section of their four-compartment stomach that ferments and digests food. These animals chew their cud and "ruminate." We humans tend to gulp and go. Unlike humans, cows are able to digest and derive energy from fibrous materials such as corn cobs and husks. And they eat balanced meals every day...no weekend binges or cheating on their diets. What the nutritionist says, goes. Cows don't jump on the scales every morning, either.

So how do you know if your, uh, clients, are getting enough to eat? I ask.

"We read the bunk," she says, assuming I understand what that means. "When we feed, we want to see about half the cows eating from the feed trough (the "bunk") and half of them sitting back not particularly hungry. Our goal is for them to eat enough but not gorge themselves."

Good idea, I say. Now tell me about corn.

"A well-balanced ration that contains corn meets 80 percent of a cow's protein needs," daughter says over the roar of the feed truck. "Corn with alfalfa hay which is high in calcium is an almost perfect diet. We call it the 'John Deere' ration. Get it? Yellow corn, green alfalfa..the color of a John Deere tractor?"

Got it; so what about grass-fed beef?

"All beef is grass-fed," she says, as if this is not the first time she has answered this question. "Most beef cattle spend 80 to 90 percent of their lives on grass (pasture) and finish their last 130 days on hay and grains such as corn or wheat, depending on where they live in the world. Animals not raised for beef, such as mother cows and bulls, are on grass all their lives. Technically, beef can be labeled 'grass-fed' if no more than 10 percent of their rations come from nutritionally concentrated cereal grains."

"Grass-finished' is a more accurate term for beef cattle that remain on grass more than 90 percent of their lives," she continues. "It takes one or two years longer to finish beef cattle this way, so these animals are older. Actually, a study was done that found the efficiency of our finishing system here in the United States results in less green house emissions and fewer forests cut down."

Interesting. What about the quality of beef? I ask. Has it changed over the past 20 years?

"It's much, much leaner," she says. "In the past, cattle were fed to become overly fat. We don't want that now. Cows today have more muscle and less fat. So today we have fewer cows that produce more beef."

CONFUSING CONTROVERSIES

FASTING AND DETOX DIETS

A patient asked me to comment on a popular "detox" diet that starts the first seven to ten days with a concoction of lemon juice, maple syrup, water and cayenne pepper, topped off with salt water and a laxative tea. Will it help me lose weight? he asked.

I'm sure it will. Any diet that withholds food and calories forces the body to feed off its own stores of energy. In this case, it's called starvation. According to a 2008 article in *Today's Dietitian*, there is little, if any, practical research on detoxifying diets. Randomized double-blind placebo-controlled studies are expensive. So why, when book sales are brisk, would one go to the trouble to actually research these diets?

Cynicism aside, fasting or withholding food or liquids for periods of time, has been used for centuries to cleanse or purify the body. Diets of clear liquids such as tea, broth, gelatin, and clear juice are often prescribed when tummies are sick and need a rest.

Flushing the bowels may feel powerful, but the body actually rids itself of harmful substances through two well-designed detoxification systems:

- Master Detox Unit, known as the "liver," is a high-tech recycling plant and the body's most active organ. Alcohol, harmful chemicals, toxic metals and other substances deemed unsafe are shuttled to the liver to be processed and removed from the body.

- Water Purification Plants, also called kidneys, continuously filter waste and toxins out of the blood and excrete them through the urine.

Adherents to detox diet plans reason that harmful chemicals "get stuck in cells" and can be cleaned out with a special diet. Whatever...but the liver and kidneys do the brunt of this work. It is true that some toxic substances are stored in fat cells; and these toxins are released when these cells are broken down and used for energy. Any weight loss diet will do that.

Are detox diets harmful? Probably not in the short term for people in good health, say most experts. Side effects, however, include diarrhea, food cravings, tiredness and headaches. And not surprising, severe restrictions of nutrients and calories over the long term can lead to life-threatening imbalances. In this case, malnutrition can be toxic, too.

NITRATES AND NITRITES

A woman tells me, "You say one thing about nutrition. Other people say something else. It makes me just want to pull a towel over my head and forget about it all."

I hear you. Not everything can be explained in a sound bite or headline. Here's a case in point: We know that a diet rich in vegetables can lower blood pressure and improve heart function. But now we know that some of these positive health effects may be due to nitrate.

Stop the presses. Aren't nitrates the substances used to cure meat products that we are supposed to avoid? Yes and no. According to an excellent review article by registered dietitian and fitness expert Ellen Coleman, nitrate is found in all vegetables and is especially abundant in beetroot (beets) and leafy greens such as spinach. Several clinical studies have found that supplementing the diet with about two cups of nitrate-rich beetroot juice each day not only lowered blood pressure but enhanced athletic performance; it did this by reducing the body's need for oxygen during exercise.

It makes sense. Dietary nitrate is converted in the body to *nitrite* which is then converted to *nitric oxide*. Nitric oxide is a good guy that regulates blood pressure and muscle function among other benefits. Thus, says Coleman, nitrate-rich foods are a source of beneficial nitric oxide that can potentially improve blood flow and enhance our physical activities.

Salts from nitrate and nitrite such as sodium nitrate and potassium nitrite are used in strictly controlled amounts to preserve food. And that's where the confusion begins. Inorganic nitrate (found naturally in beets, spinach, celery and nitrate salts) is nontoxic. But inorganic *nitrite* (found in some dietary supplements) may cause serious harm in relatively low doses. In fact, nitrite toxicity can be lethal.

Another note of caution. Organic nitrate and nitrite is not the same as food that is grown "organically." For example, organic nitrate is an ingredient in the potent heart drug *nitroglycerine*. "Any confusion that could lead to a large unintentional intake of organic nitrates or nitrites is potentially life threatening," warns Coleman.

On the other hand, research has shown that a daily intake of 300 to 500 milligrams of *dietary* nitrate (what is found in food) can improve exercise performance and lower blood pressure. Two cups of beetroot juice, for example, contains about 500 milligrams of dietary nitrate. One-half cup of raw spinach contains 450 milligrams of nitrates. And a half cup of cooked collard greens contains 200 milligrams.

Finally, one harmless but sometimes alarming side effect of eating beets: Pigments that make beets red can turn urine that color, too. Not to worry; this too will pass.

REFLECTION: Nitrate (NO_3) and nitrite (NO_2) have long been used in the preservation of meat, according to a 2013 review on this topic in the Journal of the Academy of Nutrition and Dietetics. In the curing process, nitrate is converted to nitrite which then converts to nitric oxide (NO). These compounds stabilize color and protect meat from Clostridium botulinum, the deadly botulism bacteria.

Animal studies suggest that nitrate and nitrite may be linked to cancer in humans. Yet other research shows that the conversion of dietary nitrate and nitrite to nitric oxide is beneficial to our heart and cardiovascular system. What can we do with this apparent paradox of nitrates being both harmful and healthful? We need more research, says registered dietitian nutritionist Eleese Cunningham, who reviewed this topic. "For those wishing to increase their nitrate intake for health benefits," she says, "it is best to obtain it from nitrate-rich vegetables like leafy greens or the roots of plants with leafy greens, such as beets."

DEBATING CHOLESTEROL WITH DR. ROY

My dentist, Dr Roy, likes to argue...or should I say, discuss, nutrition topics with me. Problem is, these discussions take place while I'm flat out in a dentist chair with my mouth gaped open.

"You need cholesterol," he announced at my last visit. "If you don't have it, your brain will turn to mush." If I hadn't had a hand in my mouth, I would have acknowledged that cholesterol is indeed a component of every cell membrane, including those of our brains.

"Too little cholesterol is bad for you," he continued. Right again. Cholesterol is necessary for nerve cells and sex hormones, to name a couple of its important functions.

"So, if cholesterol is so important, we should eat more of it." If my mouth hadn't been cranked open, I would have disagreed. Our bodies can make all the cholesterol we need. All creatures that have a liver can manufacture cholesterol, even if they never eat a bite of it in their food. Cows, for example, eat cholesterol-free

Quinn-Essential Nutrition

vegetarian diets. Yet, they produce cholesterol that shows up in milk and meat.

When harmful (LDL) cholesterol builds up in the blood, more is available to dig into the walls of the arteries, I rehearse to myself as Roy digs in my mouth. Over time, with more cholesterol in the arteries, the heart has to work harder to push blood through narrowed spaces. That, my friend, is heart disease.

"All cholesterol isn't bad." I nod my head in agreement. One beneficial cholesterol molecule is HDL which picks excess cholesterol out of the blood and recycles it back to the liver.

"But we shouldn't eat too much cholesterol," he says as he puts the finishing touches on my teeth. Indeed, but we also shouldn't eat too much saturated fat, which is the bigger culprit of high blood cholesterol. Still, saturated fat is often paired with cholesterol in high-fat meat, butter, cream and cheese.

"That does it," Dr. Roy says to me as he takes off my bib and sits me up in the chair. "You're out of here."

Gee...my mouth is sore. Was it something I said?

REFLECTION: Dr. Roy continues to keep me open-mouthed with his latest news on nutrition. And my teeth don't look so bad either.

CARDIOLOGIST RESPONSE TO CHOLESTEROL AND COCONUT OIL

A letter that arrived from a medical student needed an expert response. So I contacted Dr. Terrance Moran, a Board Certified Cardiologist and Lipidologist (expert in the study of fats). Moran is the Director of the Advanced Lipid Management Program at Community Hospital of the Monterey Peninsula and is an Associate Clinical Professor at the University of California in San

Francisco. I asked for his comments (and added my additions in parentheses). Hang onto your hat.

Med student: "It is becoming apparent that the things we've been told the last 40 years that cause heart disease probably aren't the culprits. Inflammation is at the root of heart disease, and cholesterol is something we can't live without. Cholesterol...is at the scene of the crime when they open up the arteries on autopsy, but it isn't the culprit. Evidence is pointing to sugar, refined carbohydrates, excess calcium supplements, and inflammatory vegetable oils...that create free radicals and oxidation when heated. The fact that 50% of heart attacks occur in people with 'normal' cholesterol is basically enough to prove the cholesterol theory false. The cholesterol myth and development of statin drugs is one of the worst falsehoods perpetuated on people in this world."

Dr. Moran: "You are partially right. A lot of people who have heart attacks do have normal lipid (cholesterol) levels. Some of this is because we usually measure the total LDL cholesterol and not the LDL "particle number" which is a much better marker of risk. The big reason for the discrepancy is that it is not primarily cholesterol that causes (heart) disease. It is a number of factors which are best summed up by genetics and the function of the endothelial cells (which line the arteries), response to inflammation, oxidative stress, and many other things.

"These basically make it more or less likely that cholesterol will accumulate in the wall of the arteries. If you have bad genetics, cholesterol will accumulate. And the higher your cholesterol, the more likely it will build up.

"So even if you have a great LDL cholesterol level, with bad genetics, the LDL is still going to accumulate. On the other hand, if you have good genetics, even with a high cholesterol, you may have little if any LDL accumulation in the arterial wall. This is why looking at someone's "lipid profile" (cholesterol numbers) is a very poor way to estimate their risk.

Quinn-Essential Nutrition

"Now all that said, it is still the LDL (cholesterol) getting into the artery wall that results in plaque (the gunk that blocks arteries). Once it gets in and stays, it becomes oxidized and sets off an inflammatory response. How aggressive that response is will be in part determined by genetics.

"We can't change our genetics but we can reduce the LDL cholesterol in our blood. Even if there are bad genetics, reducing LDL makes less of it available to get into the wall and develop into plaque. This is why the statin trials have been beneficial. Numerous studies have shown that aggressively lowering LDL cholesterol can cause plaque to regress.

"I agree that sugar and refined carbohydrates play a huge role in (heart) disease. But much of that is through their effect on lipids (fats called triglycerides) in patients with insulin resistance (those with pre-diabetes or type 2 diabetes).

"For example, high blood levels of triglycerides usually indicate smaller (more dangerous) LDL particles in the blood. And how many of these particles can burrow into the walls of the arteries and set off the inflammatory response is genetically determined."

Student: "From my research, coconut is one of the healthiest foods on this planet, judging from the millions of people whose dietary fat consists mainly of coconut, and their low incidence of heart problems."

Dr. Moran: "Before you rest on coconut as the oil of choice, please review the (medical) literature. How many studies compare a coconut-oil based diet to other diets in terms of reducing cardiovascular disease? Probably none. Yet numerous studies show the Mediterranean diet supplemented with olive oil significantly reduces cardiovascular risk and cancer. And this diet has been touted as the closest diet to what our ancestors were genetically designed for."

Barbara A. Quinn, MS, RD, CDE

REFLECTION: It's never too late to adopt a Mediterranean eating style, say experts. A long-term study reported in the September 2013 issue of the Journal of the American Medical Association Internal Medicine analyzed the diets of healthcare workers who had suffered a heart attack. Those who adopted a diet high in whole grains, fruits and vegetables and low in trans fats, meat, and sugary drinks were 40 percent less likely to die of heart disease.

ARE MILK DRINKERS BIG BABIES?

I read with interest an opinion piece that implied milk drinkers are big babies. Let me say this about that: It is true we humans are the only mammals who drink milk past infancy. We are also the only mammals who drink Starbucks on our way to work.

Some suggest we let nature steer our decisions about what we eat...and remember that other animals do not drink milk past infancy. Which makes me wonder, if horses eat hay and tigers track down other animals and tear them to shreds for dinner, should we do the same? And no, we humans do not drink our mother's milk past childhood; yet we make food from the milk of other animals. Is this a problem?

"There is a long historical and archaeological history of human use of milk in the Central Sahara (desert) based on paintings made by stone-age humans dating to 3500 to 4000 B.C," writes Dr. Louis Grivetti, noted nutrition researcher and professor emeritus of the University of California at Davis.

He explains that within societies of humans that traditionally milk animals for food, the ability to digest milk is sustained throughout adulthood. East Africans, for example, can digest fresh milk easily. People from West Africa, where milk is not a staple food, cannot do so.

Quinn-Essential Nutrition

Is it true only a few humans on the planet continue to drink milk and they are mostly Caucasians (white people)? "There are millions of people globally who are *not* Caucasians who are able to digest milk," states Grivetti. And, he adds, "most of the animals that are milked in the world are sheep and goats, not cows."

"Further," he continues, "statements that there is no science, health benefit, or examples in nature to justify milk for adults is patently false. Yes, humans get some forms of calcium from plants but in many plant foods the calcium is bound and not available for absorption."

He's right. Solid research shows that calcium from milk or supplements increases the density of bones. It builds skeletons and teeth. Dairy calcium has also been shown to lower blood pressure and may help prevent colon cancer.

The point is this: Milk is a significant source of essential nutrients, most notably calcium and protein, that are necessary for human health and longevity. Dairy foods are not the only sources of these nutrients, however. Calcium is also found in beans, broccoli, spinach and kale. Milk just happens to be the most abundant and easily absorbed source of calcium in our diet.

Still, there are those who cannot or choose not to eat or drink dairy foods. And this is America. We are free to choose what we eat...or not. Let's not be big babies about it.

REFLECTION: A small observational study reported in 2015 in the American Journal of Clinical Nutrition, found that older adults with greater intakes of dairy foods had higher levels of glutathione in their brains. Glutathione is an antioxidant that may help preserve aging brain tissue from the effects of oxidative stress. Dairy foods, these authors noted, seem to be a good source of the building materials needed by the brain to produce glutathione.

Barbara A. Quinn, MS, RD, CDE

WHEAT BELLY

I was happily munching a slice of warm bread placed on the table by our attentive waiter. Nearby, I overheard a gentleman explain to his companion that he does not eat bread...or anything else that contains wheat.

"Do you have celiac disease?" his friend inquired. (People with celiac disease cannot digest gluten, a protein in wheat, rye and barley.)

"No," he said. "But I felt much better when I stopped eating wheat." He then began to describe a book he had read on the topic. I munched a bit slower to hear the name of the book. *Wheat Belly,* by William Davis, MD, describes "wheatlessness" as "the happy, healthy state achieved by not eating wheat." Davis sees wheat as a "chronic poison" and recommends a wheat-free diet for everyone. And he makes some interesting claims to back up his distain for this grain.

Davis states that the wheat we eat today is not the wheat of 1950 or 1960. That is true, says food chemist Julie Jones, who compared statements in Davis' book to current scientific evidence in *Cereal Foods World, a* publication of international grain researchers. "Modern cultivated food plants are the product of plant breeding," Jones states, "and wheat is no exception."

Davis' book also states that today's wheat is a "modern creation of genetics research." Au contraire, says Jones. Agronomist Norman Borlaug, considered by many to be the father of the Green Revolution, won the Nobel Peace Prize in 1970 for using traditional plant breeding techniques to produce higher yields of grains (including wheat) that were better suited to their environment. Wheat remains one of the few crops in the United States that is *not* produced by genetic biotechnology.

Davis claims today's wheat crops are dangerous hybrids of unique proteins with destructive properties. Hybridization, or crossing two different varieties of wheat, does not create unique proteins, says Jones. Plants can only express proteins from their DNA code.

Eliminate wheat and you'll lose weight, says Davis. (He also frowns on corn, potatoes, rice and gluten-free foods.) Yes, you will probably lose weight if you eliminate these foods. You will also lose weight if you cut out any significant source of calories in your diet.

Interesting too, says Jones, that gluten, the protein in wheat, can stimulate hormones that tell your brain you are not hungry. In fact, she says, some data suggest that consumption of proteins such as gluten may be a good dietary strategy for weight management.

We go through "wheat withdrawal" when we give up wheat, says Davis, because of addictive opiates produced when we digest wheat protein. To which Massachusetts psychiatrist Emily Deans, MD, responds: "Wheat, we know, has breakdown components... which activate the opiate receptors in the brain and nervous system This...is part of the reward pathway. And it is activated by anything 'rewarding' including sex, exercise, drugs, gambling, and rock and roll."

Still, it is true that any person diagnosed with celiac disease, gluten intolerance, or wheat allergy must avoid wheat in all forms. Those with celiac disease or gluten sensitivity must also avoid rye and barley. But let's not ignore facts from reliable research that support significant health benefits for folks who eat whole grains, including wheat, on a regular basis. Whole grain foods have been shown to lower our risk for heart disease, cancer, diabetes, and obesity.

Should we believe that wheat is "the world's most destructive dietary ingredient"? Perhaps we should ask an entire nation of vibrant pasta-eating Italians. And as we think about ways to lose weight, Jones reminds us that "weight loss diets with the greatest long-term success rates are those that include *all* the food groups, only in smaller amounts."

I'd say that's worth chewing on.

Barbara A. Quinn, MS, RD, CDE

> *REFLECTION: Dr. Jones' analyses of selected statements from* Wheat Belly *was also published by the American Association of Cereal Chemists International (AACCI), a global nonprofit organization of nearly 2,500 scientists and professionals who study the chemistry of cereal grains.*

CLAIMS AND FACTS ABOUT RASPBERRY KETONES

Wouldn't it just be wonderful if a pill could instantly dissolve away our unwanted pounds? Some claim to have found it in a supplement called Raspberry Ketone. Others warn us to look at the facts. Here's what we know about raspberry ketone, thanks to some smart investigation by registered dietitian Marian Crockett:

Claim: "Raspberry ketone is the primary aroma compound of red raspberries."

Fact: This is true. Raspberry ketone (also referred to as RK) is a chemical compound that gives raspberries their fruity fragrance. Food and cosmetic manufacturers add it to their products for this purpose.

Claim: "Research has shown that raspberry ketone can help with weight loss efforts, especially when paired with regular exercise and a well-balanced diet of healthy and whole foods."

Fact: Regular exercise and a well-balanced diet do indeed help with weight loss efforts. Raspberry ketone has not been scientifically studied in humans, so it's anyone's guess if it aids weight loss or not.

Claim: "Raspberry ketone causes the fat within your cells to get broken up more effectively, helping your body burn fat faster."

Fact: Perhaps if you are a rat. One study tested RK on 6 obese male rats and compared it to 6 other rats. The rats fed RK were more likely to lose weight. Another study exposed RK to fat cells in a test tube and found that RK stimulated the breakdown of these cells.

Claim: "The recommended dose of raspberry ketone for weight loss is 100 milligrams per day."

Fact: Who knows? No human studies have yet been done. (I think I already said this.) If we extrapolate the dosage given in the six-obese-male-rat study to humans, it would translate to several thousand milligrams a day.

Claim: "Raspberry ketone products are made from ingredients that are 100 percent natural, ensuring that there are no negative side effects."

Fact: Rattlesnakes are 100 percent natural and can still bite you. Some concern has been expressed that RK is chemically similar to a stimulant called "synephrine" which can increase heart rate and blood pressure; this is not a good idea for anyone with heart issues.

Claim: RK "slices up fat molecules so they burn easier."

Fact: RK's chemical structure is similar to capsaicin, the heat-generating substance in hot peppers. In a test tube, RK appears to stimulate a protein that breaks down fat.

Claim: "Raspberry ketone is a miracle fat burner in a bottle."

Fact: Raspberry ketone is a "miracle money maker" in a bottle. Unless you are an obese male rat, it is way to early to draw any conclusions about the effectiveness or safety of RK as a weight loss aid.

In 2013, a review article in the *International Journal of Sports Nutrition* concluded: "There is no strong research evidence indicating that a specific supplement will produce significant weight loss, especially in the long term. Weight-loss supplements containing metabolic stimulants (such as caffeine, ephedra, or synephrine) are most likely to produce adverse side effects and should be avoided."

SCIENCE OF GMO'S

I never dreamed that the science of food and nutrition would become such hot topics in our culture. Case in point is the current battle over whether or not to require a special label on food produced with genetic engineering.

GMO (Genetically Modified Organism) is a term used for a plant that has had its genetic code partially changed in order to produce one with improved traits. Other terms that denote this type of biotechnology include "genetic engineering" or "transgenic" technology.

Biotechnology has been used in over 40 species of plants in the past two decades, according to the USDA Agricultural Research Service. Some crops, such as corn and cotton, have been genetically modified to resist insects which lessens the need for insecticides. Other foods crops have been developed with increased or improved nutrient contents.

Interestingly, a common product that is produced by genetic engineering is human insulin. People with type 1 diabetes lack the ability to produce this hormone naturally and therefore must inject this life-saving medication into their bodies several times a day.

In the process of studying crops and other substances produced through biotechnology, however, some have raised concerns that we are playing with Mother Nature in a way that is not natural. Which begs the question, Is "natural" always safe and "biotechnology" always bad? Ask someone who accidentally ate a poisonous mushroom; or consider a child in a developing country who dies before the age of five because of a diet that lacked essential nutrients that could have been provided through bio-fortified foods.

Are foods produced with genetic engineering techniques better, or worse, than traditional crops? An evidence-based study commissioned by the World Health Organization (WHO) found potential health benefits and risks with the use of foods produced through biotechnology.

As for the debate regarding labels for GMO foods, I most agree with this sensible statement that appeared in the *Santa Maria Times*, a newspaper in the small farming community of Santa Maria, California:

"California is noted nationally for the high-quality produce grown by our farmers. These vegetables and strawberries are sold nationally in many states. If each state were to enact its own food-labeling requirement, producers could have as many as 50 different labeling requirements, depending upon which state the crop was destined for.

"There would be a cost associated with managing these different labels, and it would burden the marketing of crops destined for interstate shipment. Farmers believe food-labeling laws should be addressed nationally, not at the state or local level. While we sympathize with consumers who are concerned about knowing what they eat, they can select produce labeled as "Certified Organic" to avoid genetically engineered crops."

That is true. Consumers can already know that their food was not produced with genetically modified seeds simply by choosing foods sold as "organic." So until we figure out whether biotechnology is an innovative way to sustain our food supply or a vast conspiracy of corporate greed, I agree with University of California at Berkeley biologist Michael Eisen who says, "When public policy intersects with science, we have a responsibility to understand the science."

Barbara A. Quinn, MS, RD, CDE

REFLECTION: *To date, no national or international agency has found evidence that foods produced by genetic engineering are metabolized by the body any differently from any other type of food. And according to the American Association for the Advancement of Science, genetically engineered foods are "the most extensively tested crops ever added to our food supply."*

Peggy G. Lemaux, PhD plant biologist at the University of California at Berkeley shared these facts at a recent meeting on this topic: For over 50 years, organic farmers have used a powdered form of Bacillus thuringiensis, a beneficial bacterium that resides naturally in the soil, to help their crops resist attacks by Lepidopteron caterpillars. These helpful bacteria are also known as "B.t." Through biotechnology, a gene from this organism can be added directly into corn plants so that every seed grows into a plant naturally immune to this caterpillar. This helps farmers grow healthier crops with fewer chemical pesticides.

Monarch butterflies are closely related to the insects that B.t. protects against, however. Yet, said Lemaux, a study which reported harm to Monarchs by B.t. pollen was under laboratory conditions. In real life, scientists question whether Monarch larvae would be exposed to this bacteria any more than they are now. According to the Institute of Food Technologists, "The traditional method of applying B.t. powder to plants poses a greater threat to Monarchs than B.t. corn produced by biotechnology."

"There are a lot of issues out there, and it is not always black and white," Lemaux noted. But as a scientist who has spent her life studying these issues, she reminds us that DNA (genetic material) resides in all living things and we eat it every day. A banana, for example, contains 50 milligrams of banana DNA "and we don't look like bananas."

Remember too, that DNA, the genetic code found in the cells of all living organisms, is a protein. And whether protein comes from eggs, fish or genetically produced soybeans, it is digested by the body. And by the way, Dr. Lemaux said she uses the term "genetically engineered" (GE) instead of "genetically modified organisms" (GMO). Why? "Because," she said, "everything is genetically modified."

FACTS ABOUT HIGH FRUCTOSE CORN SYRUP

Perhaps we should have paid more attention in our college chemistry classes. It would have been helpful in our understanding of high fructose corn syrup and its effects on health. Case in point: The respected Center for Science in the Public Interest (CSPI) sent a letter to the major of San Francisco opposing his proposal to tax beverages made with high fructose corn syrup, but excluding drinks made with other forms of sugar. Scientific evidence, they said, shows that high fructose corn syrup has no more detrimental effect on health than does regular sugar. How can this be? Let's put on our chemistry goggles and consider these facts:

High Fructose Corn Syrup (HFCS) is a sweetener made from corn. Corn kernels contain corn starch which are molecules of glucose connected in long chains. Enzymes similar to those in our bodies that digest food are used to break these long chains into individual glucose molecules to make corn syrup. Other enzymes then convert about half the glucose in corn syrup to the sugar, fructose. Thus "high fructose corn syrup" was so-named because it is higher in fructose than regular corn syrup.

HFCS is as sweet as sucrose (table sugar). But HFCS is more stable and less expensive to make than sugar from cane or beets; that's why it shows up in everything from sodas to spaghetti sauce.

High fructose corn syrup is chemically similar to sugar (sucrose). Sucrose, or "table sugar" is refined from sugar cane or beets and is 50 percent fructose and 50 percent glucose. High fructose corn syrup can be either 42 percent fructose and 58 percent glucose (which technically could be called "low fructose corn syrup") or 55 percent fructose and 45 percent glucose, which is very similar to sugar.

Sugar, honey and HFCS are digested the same. Really. Sugar is broken down in the body to fructose and glucose. Honey is digested to fructose and glucose, as is HFCS.

It's the fructose part of sugar and HFCS that has scientists worried. Large amounts of fructose (in the absence of glucose) may interfere with the body's ability to metabolize fats and may be related to our growing obesity problem.

Fructose does have some redeeming qualities. It is the primary sugar in fruit. It is less likely to cause tooth decay than other sugars. It does not raise blood sugar levels or stimulate insulin to the same extent as other types of sugar. And fructose is the main component of "fructans," health-promoting substances in fruits and vegetables that feed the good bacteria in our gut. Fructooligosaccharides (FOS) and inulin are two examples of these beneficial compounds.

Too much of *any* sugar can lead to health problems. Consider that a cup of apple juice contains the same amount of fructose as a cup of soda sweetened with HFCS. And agave syrup has a *higher* percentage of fructose than HFCS. If we avoid products with high fructose corn syrup and choose ones loaded with other sugars instead, we've missed a very important point. "The real issue," states the *Center for Science in the Public Interest*, "is that excessive consumption of any sugars may lead to health problems."

REFLECTION: An article in the July 1, 2013 issue of the Journal of the American Medical Association by David S. Ludwig, MD, PhD reviews the health effects of common sugars in our diet which are primarily mixtures of fructose and glucose. Based on the current evidence, Dr. Ludwig recommends that we reduce our intake of all highly processed sugars, not just fructose.

ESSENTIALS OF FLUORIDE

My mom never had cavities and now she's got more than her fair share. What happened? She has a medical condition that prevents her mouth from making adequate amounts of saliva, the fluid that bathes teeth with nutrients and other substances to protect them from decay.

Fluoride is one of those nutrients and thus is an essential trace mineral, according to a position paper on this topic by the *Academy of Nutrition and Dietetics*. In other words, fluoride is a mineral required by the body in teeny-tiny, or trace amounts. In teeth and bones, fluoride works from the inside out. It helps stabilize other minerals like calcium and phosphorous in these structures. And fluoride is one of only a few known substances that can stimulate the growth of bone cells.

Before teeth erupt in the mouth, fluoride fortifies tooth enamel so it can resist cavities. And continuous exposure to fluoride after teeth are formed prevents bacteria from eroding tooth surfaces. That's the reason for fluoridated toothpaste and those fluoride swishes your dentist springs on you during dental check-ups.

Like many trace nutrients, however, there is a fine line between enough and too much fluoride. Just one part fluoride per million in drinking water is enough to protect teeth from cavities.

Excess amounts of more than 1 milligram a day for infants or 10 milligrams a day for older children and adults, can be toxic and cause irreversible stains or "mottling" on the teeth. Here then, are some guidelines for the use of fluoride from nutrition and dental experts:

- Know if your water supply if fluoridated. (About two-thirds of the public water in the United States contains fluoride.) Well water varies in fluoride content.
- Besides drinking water, find out how much fluoride you might be ingesting in your diet. Tea and fish, for example, can be significant sources of dietary fluoride. You can find a complete list of the fluoride content of foods at www.ars.usda.gov/SP2UserFiles/Place/80400525/Data/Fluoride/F02.pdf
- Follow your dentist's advice regarding supplemental fluoride. Because the risk for mottled teeth is highest in younger children, the *American Dental Association* does not recommend the use of fluoride toothpaste or fluoride mouth rinses for unsupervised children under the age of six years.
- Don't swallow your toothpaste. Fluoride toothpaste works best on the surface of teeth.
- Teach kiddos to use no more than a pea-size amount of toothpaste when they brush.

Not everyone is happy about adding fluoride to public water supplies. Based on decades of research and observation however, arguments against the use of water fluoridation are unfounded, say dental experts. Remember too, that fluoride is a natural element of soil and water. When used and consumed properly, it is safe and extremely beneficial to the integrity of bones and teeth. Just remember that a little goes a long way.

REFLECTION: After a review of the most current evidence, the Academy of Nutrition and Dietetics reaffirmed its position that fluoride is a beneficial nutrient. This professional organization stated, "The use of fluorides for the prevention of dental caries is recognized as the most effective dental public health measure in existence. Fluoride is beneficial to all age groups throughout the life cycle."

The United States Centers for Disease Control and Prevention (CDC) named the fluoridation of water as one of the ten most important public health measures of the twenty-first century. As of 2013, almost 75 percent of Americans were served by community water systems enriched with fluoride.

DOSE MAKES THE POISON

A patient once told me his leukemia (a type of cancer) was being treated with a low dose of arsenic. Wait. Isn't arsenic a…POISON? It is in high doses; but arsenic is also a trace element that may be beneficial in micro (itty bitty) amounts.

I like to add nutmeg to my oatmeal cookie dough. It's a wholesome spice, right? Yet in high doses (more than five grams or a teaspoonful) nutmeg can be toxic, according to case reports from the National Toxicology Program of the US Department of Health and Human Services.

"The dose makes the poison," says toxicologist Carl Winter, who works with the Food Science and Technology program at the University of California at Davis. Winter is also a leading authority on the use of pesticides in food. "It is the amount of a chemical rather than its presence or absence that determines the potential for harm," says Winters.

Most plants for example, produce natural toxins that help protect them from mold, fungus and insects. Our food contains

10,000 times more of these natural pesticides than the synthetic variety applied by farmers, says Winter; yet they are not concentrated enough to be dangerous. Residues of pest-fighting substances on plants are measured in parts per billion (PPB). One part per billion is like 1 second in 32 years, he says. So whether or not a detectable residue of a pesticide constitutes a health hazard depends on the amount. High doses of anything, including medications, vitamins, and x-rays, can be harmful, says Winter. This is the method used by scientists to determine what is safe:

Step One: Measure the highest amount of a substance that can be given to an animal before a negative effect is seen. That is the "Maximum Tolerated Dose" and is usually thousands of times higher than what is normally present in our food.

Step Two: Determine what dose at which that same substance causes *no* effect on laboratory animals. This is the "No Observable Effect Level."

Step Three: Lower the No Observable Effect Level (from Step 2) another 100 to 1000 times; and add additional safety margins for infants and children. This is the "Acceptable Daily Intake," the maximum dose that can safely be allowed in one day. Because of these strict standards, the actual amounts of detectable residues we ingest are generally less than one percent of the Acceptable Daily Intake, says Winter.

Of course we want healthier alternatives for controlling pests that threaten our food. And so do farmers, since they eat their food, too. Here are some ideas from food safety experts:

1. **Keep eating fruits and vegetables.** Evidence that shows a lower risk for cancer and other chronic diseases in people who eat more fruits and vegetables is based on typical grocery store food, not necessarily from an organic market. The benefits of eating a mostly plant-based diet far outweigh any potential risk of pesticide residues.

2. **Wash and peel produce.** Pesticide residue can be removed by washing fruit and vegetables in water, says Winter. Throw away the outer leaves of lettuce, cabbage, and other leafy vegetables.
3. **Eat a variety of foods.** Pesticide use varies from crop to crop. Eating a variety can minimize exposure to any one substance.

REFLECTION: Research studies and clinical trials found that a form of arsenic called "arsenic trioxide" was a useful treatment for certain types of leukemia. It has been approved by the US Food and Drug Administration for this use.

UNDERSTANDING PESTICIDE USE

Brian Leahy has an interesting history. In 1980, he operated a 900-acre organic rice farm in California. In the 1990's, he managed 800 acres of organic corn, soybean, alfalfa and cattle in Nebraska. In 2002, he became executive director of the California Certified Organic Farmers (CCOF). And in 2012, Leahy became the director of the California Department of Pesticide Regulations.

"Pesticides will always be part of modern life," says Leahy in a recent interview with the Alliance for Food and Farming. "I want to show people that you can effectively manage pests by using pesticides as a last resort and choosing ones that are less toxic to people."

Guess he knows what he's talking about. California produces half the vegetables, fruits and nuts (no pun intended) in the US. The Golden State also has the nation's most comprehensive program to regulate pesticide use. "Our modern food supply, public health and resource management all rely on pesticides," says Leahy.

Yep, we heard that right. As scary as the term may sound, a "pesticide" is any substance that protects our food crops from dangerous insects or microbes. Even organic farmers use pesticides, says Leahy. Most are derived from microorganisms or other natural sources; some are synthetically produced. And all are approved by the USDA National Organic Program (NOP).

Pesticides used on organic as well as conventional crops undergo the same rigorous scientific evaluation by the Environmental Protection Agency (EPA), says Leahy. This is to ensure they will not harm people when used according to label instructions.

But really, aren't organic pesticides better? Jon Marthedal, who grows conventional as well as certified organic blueberries in Fresno, California, states, "To some extent the operations are very similar. We use fungicides, fertilizers and insecticides in both operations. The big difference is the source of the chemical. When it is certified as organic, it has to be a naturally occurring organic compound. And it's interesting, because a lot of the chemicals that we use in our conventional operation are really just synthetic versions of the organic compounds that we use in our organic operations."

Soledad farmer Rod Braga grows vegetables both organically and conventionally. He states, "I think what people need to understand is that we do use pesticides on organic vegetables. And the rate at which we use them on the organic crops are actually at a much higher volume, and often, more applications than we do on the conventional side. We just wouldn't be able to produce enough crops to feed everybody if we were organically growing and not using any pesticides."

Which begs the question: Is organic healthier than conventionally grown produce? Remember, say experts with the Alliance for Food and Farming, the term "organic" defines how a food is produced. It does not address quality, safety or nutritional value.

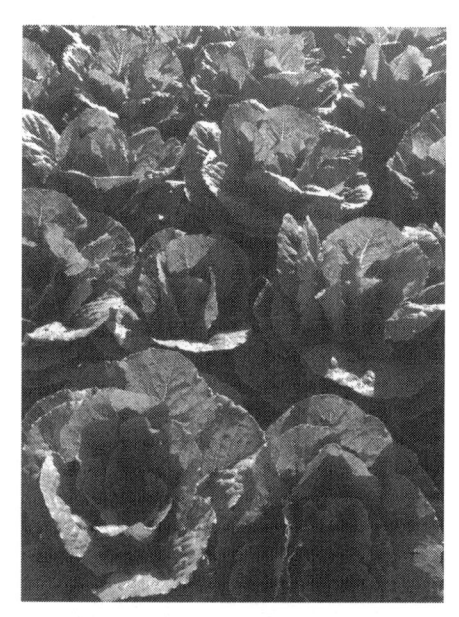

Taylor Farms lettuce field, Salinas, California

REFLECTION: A 2012 study estimated that 20,000 cancer cases per year could be prevented in the United States if half the US population increased its fruit and vegetable consumption by just one serving each day, whether from organic or conventionally grown crops.

In 2014, the British Journal of Nutrition published a review of current studies from around the world, including research in Europe, the US, Brazil, Canada and Japan. This report found significantly higher concentrations of several antioxidant compounds such as flavonoids and polyphenols in organically grown fruits and vegetables compared to those grown conventionally. This study contradicts earlier studies that found no significant differences between organic and conventional crops.

One observation continues to be true: People who eat more vegetables and fruit from a variety of sources maintain better health over the long run than those who don't.

NUTRITION FOR A LIFETIME

NUTRITION NURSERY RHYMES

It was a baby shower themed after vintage nursery rhymes, complete with Little Bo Peep and her sheep and Mary quite contrary. My daughter, pregnant with my granddaughter, sat on Miss Muffet's tuffet while a spider sat beside her, and opened her gifts.

I was curious about the food. For example, when Little Miss Muffet ate her curds and whey, what exactly was she eating? Cottage cheese most likely, say those who think about these matters. In the cheese making process, some proteins in milk clump together to form curds. Others remain in the liquid called "whey." Cottage cheese which supposedly was named for people who lived in cottages and made this simple cheese, contains curds and whey. Both are complete proteins because they contain all the amino acids needed to assemble any protein structure in the body. These complete proteins are therefore important for building babies.

Whey protein in particular is rich in leucine, an amino acid that helps synthesize muscle tissue..and not just in grand-babies. Studies show that whey protein benefits aging muscles in grand-mommies as well.

Jack and Jill ran up the hill to fetch a pail of water. Jack fell down and broke his crown and Jill gave him sips from her water bottle...or something like that. Jill knew that water is a critically important nutrient, especially during pregnancy. It is the solvent

Quinn-Essential Nutrition

and coolant for all the biochemical reactions in the baby-building process. Water also delivers necessary nutrients from pregnant moms to growing babies and carries away wastes. Pregnant mommies need to drink about ten cups of fluid from water and other beverages each day, according to current recommendations. During the months of breastfeeding, a woman need about 13 cups of fluids each day.

Humpty Dumpty sat on a wall; Humpty Dumpty had a great fall. All the King's horses and men couldn't put Humpty together again. So they cooked up some eggs which are a rich source of choline, a relatively unknown but essential nutrient for pregnancy. Choline is especially important for fetal brain development. It also helps to strengthen cell membranes and aids in memory development and cognition, the ability to think clearly. Other good sources of choline include lean beef, cauliflower and peanuts. Human milk is also a rich source of choline.

Now about that old woman who lived in a shoe...

BASIC RULES FOR FEEDING KIDS...AND PUPPIES

Having a puppy is like...having another child. Well, not exactly. My kids never chewed on my shoes. And my puppy will never leave for college one day. But there are a few nutritional rules these youngsters have in common:

Appropriate food. Puppy chow is a balanced formula of essential protein, fat, carbohydrate, calcium, iron and other nutrients needed for this time of rapid growth. Kids too, need to chow on a variety of foods so they get all the nutrients they need for proper growth and development.

Consistent feeding schedule. Puppies develop best with regular meals; so do kids. And no, puppies cannot eat at the table. But children should, as often as possible with the family. Studies on young teens find that students who dine regularly with their

Barbara A. Quinn, MS, RD, CDE

parents score better on school work and spend less time watching television.

No extreme diets. Puppies and youngsters don't do well on fat free diets. Most experts recommend whole milk until the age of two years. Lower fat foods are OK after that.

Occasional fun foods. No begging allowed. Mom and Dad should decide when and what occasions justify special treats.

Encourage activity. Puppies are happy and sleep well after a day of herding cats and playing outside. Kids too, should be involved in age-appropriate activities each day, says the *National Association for Sport and Physical Education (NASPE)*. Toddlers and preschoolers for example, should not be sedentary for more than an hour at a time except when they are sleeping, says the NASPE. Children and teens need 30 minutes to an hour of brisk play or other physical activity each day.

Set limits on television. Parents are responsible to set limits on the time their children spend viewing television and computer screens, says the *American Academy of Pediatrics (AAP)*. And since excessive television and computer time is linked to obesity in children and teens, the AAP recommends we keep our children's rooms "media-free."

Limit sodas. My puppy slurps clean water when he is thirsty. Yet today, our American children and teenagers are drinking more soft drinks—500 times more than children 50 years ago. With 150 calories and at least 10 teaspoons of sugar in each (12 ounce) can, many researchers are not surprised that the number of overweight kids in the US has more than doubled in the past 20 years.

Set a good example. Youngsters need good, not perfect, examples to follow as they grow and develop into independent individuals. Now, what happened to my other tennis shoe?

FEEDING MISS FRANCES

Dear Tom,

It's been one year since you became a father. And in my opinion, your daughter (my granddaughter) is the most perfect child in the world. Frances, who is named after her great-grandmother, is not the biggest apple in the basket; neither is she the smallest. She is perfectly healthy for her God-given size.

And besides good genes and you as her daddy, Frances is blessed with a mommy who feeds her very sensibly. Stephanie calmly offers little princess a variety of foods at appropriate intervals during the day. And because of that, Frances is happy and trusting and eats what she needs when she is hungry. In the words of Mr. Rogers (remember him?), "Knowing deep within us that someone is going to feed us when we are hungry is how trust and love begin."

Child nutrition experts agree. According to "the feeding doctor," Katia Rowell, MD, *how* we feed our children is as important as *what* we feed them. We can unwittingly set our kids up for what she calls "weight dysregulation" when we worry too much about how they eat. Rowell calls it the "worry cycle" that can lead to food struggles and disordered eating habits.

Your goal as a parent? Raise little Frances to become a competent eater, someone who eats a variety of foods and can decide when she is hungry and when she is not. Competent eaters have better nutrition, enjoy food in a healthier way, and tend to thrive better socially and emotionally, say experts.

Here are some other recommendations from child feeding authorities:

Know the division of responsibilities. Parents are responsible for what, where, and when their youngster eats, says registered dietitian and child feeding author, Ellyn Satter. Children are responsible for how much they eat of kid-appropriate food. (No pretzels or beer, please.)

Move toward structure. Kids do not need to graze like horses or cattle. Miss Frances need to sit down for appropriately spaced meals and snacks, or about every two to three hours for most young children.

Eat meals together as a family. As she observes others, Frances is more apt to try new foods and learn how to regulate her own intake.

Give up control. Power struggles with food can backfire, Dr. Rowell warns. A child forced to eat more may resist and eat less. And children of overly restrictive parents may be driven to eat more. Frances is capable of regulating her own food intake when she is fed in ways that preserve those skills.

Recognize cues for hunger and fullness. Like most young children, Frances gets a bit fussy when she is hungry. And when she is ready to eat, she opens her mouth freely when food is offered. When she has had enough, thank you very much, she turns her head away and closes her mouth. She's fortunate to have a dad and mom who recognize those important signals.

Introduce new tastes along with at least one familiar food. Youngsters like Frances may need to try a new food several times (sometimes up to ten times) before she decides she likes it...or not.

Expect a mess. Little ones armed with spoons and soft foods can be alarming. But think of it this way: one small spill for Frances, one giant leap towards being a competent eater.

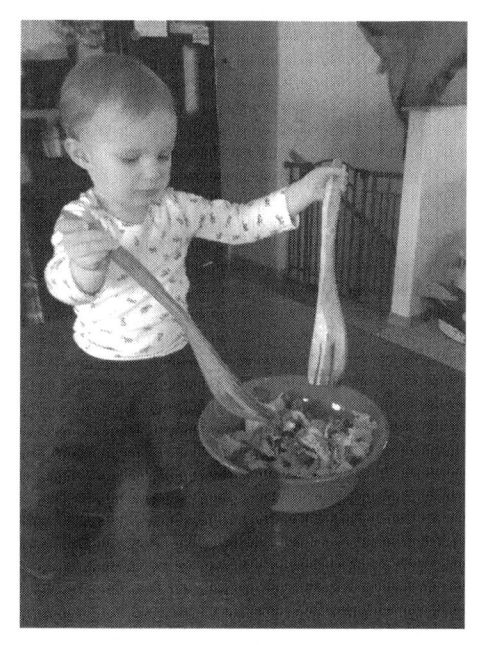

Frances Ann Furman Age 22 months

REFLECTION: My friend, Kathy became a grandmother last year and sent me this reflection on how she raised her two children on their family farm in Colusa, California:

"I followed similar guidelines with my children and they were fast learners. They never needed to stuff themselves because there was more where that came from...even a few sweets and snacks. If they wanted cookies after school, we had cookies, but in moderation.

"Also, I sent them out to play every day after school; no special toys, just play. Their favorite of all was when we were replanting trees in the orchard and their Dad had taken the bulldozer and pushed the trees out, leaving a slanting hole in the ground. They had more fun digging and running up and down and shoveling and throwing dirt clods than any fancy toys ever provided. Best of all, they were being active, getting fresh air, and exercising their imaginations. What could

possibly be better! And the fact that they had to get undressed on the back porch by the washing machine because they were so dirty, was never a problem for them or for me. After all, dirt is what paid for those clothes in the first place."

TEACHING KIDS TO EAT..BUT NOT TOO MUCH

A frantic mother called about her child's voracious appetite. "He just wants to eat all the time!" Another mom was worried that her little darling was starving. "He just doesn't eat enough!"

So, how do we entice little ones to eat...but not too much? Start by realizing that is not our job, says registered dietitian and psychotherapist Ellyn Satter. In her book, *Secrets of Feeding a Heathy Family*, Satter explains that parents just need to provide reasonable meals and snacks at reasonable times; that's all.

Really? Except in rare genetic disorders, kids are born with the ability to eat the right amount of food for their own bodies, Satter reassures. If we try to over-control how much they eat, little ones can lose their "internal food regulation mechanism," a complex system that tells them when they need to eat and when they are satisfied with enough food.

How can we encourage this natural process? Reinforce what your children intuitively know about how to eat, advises Satter. "The goal is not to try to change the way a child eats, but to help your child be more aware of what goes on inside of him." Here are some of her suggestions:

Help children appreciate how they look. Every body is different. And part of growing up, says Satter, is coming to terms with what nature has provided.

Teach kids to recognize body signals related to eating. And understand these terms yourself:

"Hunger" is how the body reminds us to eat. True hunger makes the stomach growl; it might make us grouchy or give us a headache. If we ignore hunger signals, our body gets confused about what and how much to eat.

"Appetite" is what we feel when we see, smell, or think about food that tastes good. Sometimes our appetite tells us to eat when we are not really hungry, such as when a freshly baked chocolate chip cookie beckons right after we have eaten a satisfying meal.

"Famished" was described by Jack Nicholson in an old western movie: "I'm so hungry, I could eat a frozen dog." Not a good idea; when we wait too long to eat, we eat too much, too fast.

"Satiety" is when our body senses we have had enough to eat and it's OK to stop eating. We can help children recognize this.

"Full" is when we eat past the point of feeling satisfied. Feeling full will normally make children uncomfortable.

"Stuffed" is beyond full, when our body shouts, "No more! I can't eat another bite!" Thanksgiving comes to mind.

Help kids make good choices. Research shows that most bodies feel best when they are fed sensible meals and snacks at regular intervals. We want our kids to come to meals hungry, not famished. And to eat until they are satisfied, not stuffed.

Let children decide how much they will eat. This is perhaps the toughest for concerned parents. But when we do not try to dictate how much little Johnny should eat, he is more apt to effectively regulate his intake according to his needs.

Practice what you preach. Ouch. It is true, however, that habits are easier caught than taught. And when we understand and accept our kids, they begin to understand and accept themselves, says Satter. I say Amen to that.

RECIPE FOR GRADUATING INTO LIFE

As you venture from school to your next step in life, here is a sure-fire recipe you may want to refer to from time to time:

Start with one student, pre-filled with hope and promise. Fold gently into close friends and family members. Season liberally with hugs, words of encouragement, and loving limits.

Add generous servings of raw and cooked fruit and vegetables to add glow to final product. Oranges and sweet peppers for example, are best eaten raw to retain more vitamin C. Cooking carrots and tomatoes releases more disease-fighting substances such as beta carotene and lycopene.

Blend in moderate amounts of protein from fish, lean meats, poultry, eggs, nuts, soy and dairy foods. Add fish at least twice a week to protect your student from inflammatory conditions that can lead to heart disease and other chronic diseases.

Note: For best results, use real foods in this recipe as much as possible. Research continues to show that ingredients in food work together synergistically (you're the graduate; look it up) with other ingredients. In other words, health benefits are more pronounced when this recipe is prepared with whole foods rather than pills and potions of isolated nutrients.

To maintain structural integrity to the final product, add daily servings of calcium-rich foods including low fat milk and yogurt or calcium-enriched products such as soy or juice beverages. Marinate in fresh water several times a day. Coffee, tea, juice and other low-sugar beverages may be substituted for water within reason.

Sprinkle with small amounts of nuts, seeds, and vegetable oils such as olive or canola to provide essential fats and improve glow.

Stir mixture vigorously for an hour each day. Allow to rest for 8 hours overnight.

Caution: Mixture may swell unfavorably if combined with excessive amounts of sugar or salt. Add these ingredients sparingly to taste. And skim off extra fat to help final product last longer.

Cover with reasonable expectations and allow to develop at an individual pace. Mixture may need to stew in alternating hot and cold motivations for several years before it is ready to serve. Mix with high quality teachers, counselors, and mentors until well-saturated with high ideals and strong values.

Serve with generous portions of love and blessings.

PEP GOES TO COLLEGE

Well, Pep—that's been your nickname from kindergarten when your aunt Molly thought you looked "peppy" in your pigtails—now you're a college student. And our last child to leave home.

You said, "I'll be fine." Your dad and your sister assure me, "She'll be fine." And after talking to you about your first day of classes, I can tell you are fine, indeed.

"I miss you." We miss you too, honey.

"I got up a little late so I got a bagel and some milk for breakfast." Good idea; you remember the importance of morning food to break your fast. Research has shown that young people who eat a morning meal perform better on thinking tasks that require concentration, such as college classes. Fueling your body (and your brain) before you hit your first course helps keep your mind on what you are learning. It may even help you score better on tests than your college pals who skip this important first meal of the day.

"My math teacher is really cool. He wears Hawaiian shirts and chews gum." That's great that you are paying attention in class.

"It's really hot. I'm drinking a lot of water." Good idea; extra fluid will help your body process the energy you need to walk to class and ride your bike around campus. Most people need at least a cup (8 ounces) of fluid for every 250 calories. That's about eight cups for most folks. In hot weather and with more activity, you'll need even more.

"I need to get some juice for the refrigerator in my dorm room." Maybe cranberry juice? Recent studies confirm that about a half cup (4 ounces) of cranberry juice every day might help prevent urinary tract infections.

"When are you going to send a care package?" Soon, dear; I won't forget you. And don't rely on easy fixes when you get a little down. A reliable clinical trial recently looked to see if the dietary supplement, ginseng, could improve mood in young adults. Could it make them more alert for early morning classes?

After eight weeks of taking this supplement, no psychological benefits were seen. Ginseng was no more effective in enhancing a healthy young person's mental functioning than a sugar pill. So stick with your tried and true remedies when college life gets you a little down, Pep. Call home. Get connected with people who care about you. Pray.

"There's this really cute guy in my English class." Better take your water bottle to that course. Extra fluid will help you stay cool when you overheat.

"I really like being in college." I'm glad, sweetheart. And we know you really are going to be just fine.

WORDS FOR A WISE GRADUATE

Dear Graduate,

I once heard that our education is what we remember after we forget what we learned. And like a variety of foods, our lessons come from a many sources. May you remember and be nourished by these timeless observations as you graduate into the next season of your life:

If we could give every individual the right nourishment and exercise---not too little and not too much---we would have found the safest way to health. (Hippocrates)

Never eat more than you can lift. (Miss Piggy)

Quinn-Essential Nutrition

The world is composed of givers and takers. The takers eat better, the givers sleep better. (my Aunt Bert)

Eat more of the best and less of the rest. (registered dietitian Leni Reed,)

Eat slowly, listen carefully, and love deeply. All have value. (notation from my mom)

Prepare for emergencies. Always have chocolate within walking distance. (personal experience)

Share with others a piece of your heart, not a piece of your mind. (Aunt Bert)

Never eat a burrito as big as your head. (inspired by a restaurant in Lincoln, Nebraska)

The happiest person is the one who counts his blessings as well as his calories. (Aunt Bert)

Too much of anything is not good for you. (My grandfather, Daniel Gold Hines.)

Take time to be well or you'll have to take time to be sick. (Unknown)

Better is a dry morsel and quietness with it, than a house full of feasting and strife. (Proverbs 17:1, NAS Bible)

Never, never, never give up. (Winston Churchill)

ADVICE FOR NEWLYWEDS

Dear Stephanie and Tom,

As you anticipate your wedding day, I know you must be thinking about vital matters such as nutrition. Not to worry. Your mom and soon-to-be mother-in-law and her dietitian friends are here for you with some words of advice:

Barbara A. Quinn, MS, RD, CDE

"Remember to eat something on the big day even if you are too nervous to feel hungry. It will give your brain nourishment during the ceremony so you can remember your vows!" (Janna)

"The one thing that I always hear—and it happened at my daughter's wedding—is that the bride and groom don't have time at the reception to eat. So it's nice if your caterer can pack a basket of food for the couple to have later that night." (Alvina)

"My mom and dad have been married for 50 years and every morning, my dad cuts up an apple and an orange and brings it to my mom for breakfast along with a moist napkin to wipe her hands. I am so blessed to have them as my parents." (Pamela)

"Make a point to eat at least one meal a day together; it's a tried and true way to develop healthful eating habits in preparation for the family to come." (Marilyn)

"Eating together is only partly about nutrition and mostly about connection and love, listening and sharing." (Lisa)

"Really *listen* to each other. And the second thing would be…you can never eat too many vegetables." (Michelle)

And to these wise words I would add: Nourish and season your life together with love and grace. Share your hearts as you share your meals. Eat slowly. Forgive quickly. And may God richly bless you!

LIFE LESSONS FROM ROY AND MARGE

I'd never known that two people, besides my own parents, could have such a profound effect on my life. Roy and Marge were two such people. This couple had great insight, not from studying science or research books, but from their many years of serving others. Here is some of the wisdom I learned from Roy and Marge:

"Always eat breakfast." Marge had this right. People who "break-the-fast" when they rise literally give their bodies a jump start on the day. Studies show that a meal in the morning helps the body burn about 200 calories more than folks who skip this important time to eat.

"Do activities to work up a sweat and exercises to keep muscles strengthened." Roy took up tennis lessons at the age of 90-something. And he never slowed down.

"Remember children, at every main meal have two vegetables, one that grows above the ground and one that grows below the ground." Marge told me she learned that from her mother and then used the advice with her own family. It's sound advice. Combinations such as broccoli and carrots, tomatoes and onions, and green beans and yams provide an array of colorful compounds known to guard us against cancer and heart disease.

"Sit around the table and enjoy the food together." Roy and Marge did this with their children. Now we know that children who eat meals with their families do better in school and they are more apt to develop better eating habits.

"Plan your meals color-wise." Nutrition science bears out what Marge knew intuitively. The color pigments that make greens "green," tomatoes "red," and grapes "purple" act as potent antioxidants that confer special health benefits to those who ingest them.

"Cream puffs are nice to eat once in a while!" Ahhh...another reason why I loved these two. Even dietitians admit food is more than nutrients. Food can symbolize love, friendship, and comfort. Those who do not fear food but enjoy if for physical and emotional health are the ones who are able to maintain healthful eating habits for the long term, say health experts.

"Stay involved with activities that have meaning." Amen. Roy and Marge showed by example how to live joyously for God and others. And Marge would laugh when I told her I wanted to be just like her when I grew up.

> REFLECTION: When Roy and Marge moved from California to Oregon to be near their children and grandchildren, their table continued to overflow with friends and healthful food. And they continued to bless and minister to others to the very last days of their lives.
>
> Roy stepped into eternity just shy of his 97th birthday one month before he and Marge could celebrate their 70th wedding anniversary. She joined him in Heaven at the age of 96.

PROVEN BEHAVIORS THAT ADD YEARS TO LIFE

Don't smoke. Be physically active. Drink moderately if you drink at all. Eat plenty of fruits and vegetables. Yeah, yeah we know all that. And by the way, if you practice *all four* of these behaviors regularly, it could add 14 years to your life. It's these combined daily habits that have the biggest impact on our health, say experts.

Here are the details: Researchers in the United Kingdom recruited over 20,000 healthy men and women between the ages of 45 to 79. They scored the participants' lifestyle habits and turned them loose for more than a decade. During that time, they documented those who died.

After about 11 years, health scores of the surviving participants were examined. After adjusting for several variables, such as dying from old age or getting hit by a car, the researchers reported a strong association between lifestyle behaviors and the risk for dying.

Deaths related to heart disease and stroke showed the strongest relationship; participants who smoked, skimped on exercise, fruits and vegetables, and drank more than a moderate amount of alcohol were four times as likely to die (particularly from heart disease) as those who practiced better habits. And the longer these habits were practiced, the better.

Want to see how you fare on this same health scale? Give yourself one point for each of these health behaviors you do on a regular basis:

1. I do not smoke or have a history of smoking.
2. I get at least 30 minutes of physical activity a day, either at work or at home.
3. I drink no more than one or two alcoholic drinks a day. (One drink is 4 to 5 ounces of wine, 8 to12 ounces of beer, or 1 to 1 1/2 ounce (shot) of liquor.)
4. I eat two to three cups fruits and vegetables every day.

According to this study, middle-aged people who score 0 (zero) are four times more likely to die, more often from heart disease, over an 11-year period than those who score a 4. Those who score a 2 are twice as likely to die compared to someone who scores a 4.

It's true; the *combined* effect of all our habits are significant. In other words, it's probable that a marathon runner who lives on beer and pretzels could have a shorter life span than a walker who enjoys an occasional glass of wine with a diet high in fruits and vegetables. What we do day by day counts for the long run.

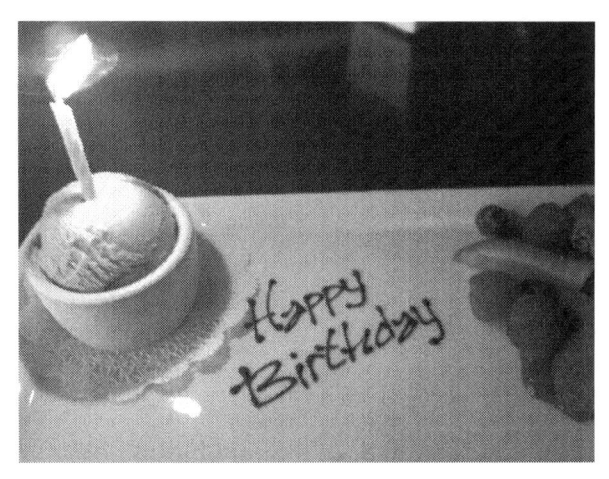

Birthday dessert at Sticks Restaurant, Pebble Beach, California

Barbara A. Quinn, MS, RD, CDE

LIVING TO 100

My aunt Bert (short for Bertha) was joyfully welcomed into heaven at the age of 101. It's amazing for me to think of her life over all those years. From what I observed, Bert truly "lived" her journey with her whole mind and body. For as long as I can remember, Bert was mentally and physically beautiful and vibrant.

How did she manage to age so gracefully? She no doubt was blessed with good genes from her parents. Researchers who study such things believe some people possess certain "longevity-enabling genes" that actually slow down the aging process and protect them from chronic diseases like diabetes and heart disease. Centenarians, people who have lived for 100 years or more generally have at least one such genetic marker.

Bert was also blessed to live in the United States, where we have the greatest number of centenarians, according the Census Bureau. (Japan has the second highest.) Bert didn't pick her genetic code; but she made other choices in her lifetime that positively contributed to her long and healthy life: She did not smoke. She enjoyed cooking and eating good food that helped keep her Audrey Hepburn-like figure. And she remained mentally and physically active most of her life.

Bert was on the go, even when she was well into her 90's. She walked; she stretched; she was a regular participant in her water aerobics class. Physical activity, say experts, help control weight and blood pressure and help prevent type 2 diabetes and osteoporosis. Being active also helps manage arthritis that can hit in later years.

Physical activity also keeps the brain popping, both cognitively and emotionally, say scientists. Activities that can significantly postpone many of the disabilities of aging include stretching, aerobic "huff and puff" exercise and strength training.

Nutritionally, Bert was never a picky eater. All her life, she enjoyed a wide variety of nourishing foods. Perhaps she had what researchers have identified as "protective nutritional factors" common to the over-100 gang. Two of these factors are high blood levels of high-density lipoprotein (HDL), a protective "good" cholesterol, and high levels of EPA and DHA, the omega-3 fatty acids found primarily in fish that protect against inflammatory diseases like heart disease and diabetes.

Centenarians have also been found to have high blood levels of antioxidant vitamin A, found in dark orange and green vegetables such as carrots and spinach, and vitamin E from whole grains, seeds, nuts and vegetable oils. Makes sense. A condition called "oxidative stress" contributes to processes that age the body. "Anti"oxidant vitamins help defend the body against oxidative stress. In fact, possibly because of the presence of these antioxidants, blood samples of long-lived folks tend to have fewer of these damaging oxidative substances.

REFLECTION: Evidence continues to show that some people have a genetic predisposition for a long life, according a 2012 update on nutrition and longevity by the Academy of Nutrition and Dietetics (AND). What influences our length of years most favorably, however, are healthful eating habits, regular physical activity, avoidance of tobacco products and a healthy body weight.

COMFORT FOOD

WHY WE EAT

Why do we eat? Sometimes we eat to fill in time, such as when the airline announced my plane was late and I may miss my connection in Phoenix. Might as well have an early lunch, I counseled myself as I headed for the comfort of the airport restaurant.

Sometimes we eat because food tastes good. "Want some?" a sparkle-eyed little boy asked as he poked his candy sucker at me from an adjoining booth. No, thank you, I smiled. "It's good!" he assured me as he stuck it back in his mouth.

Sometimes we eat because we know what we need. "French fries, potato salad, or macaroni salad with your sandwich?" the waitress asked. I considered how soon I would be in the vicinity of any vegetables that day. I asked for a tossed salad.

Sometimes we eat when things go wrong. Our connecting flight is...cancelled? For two days? Why am I suddenly digging in my purse for that little bag of M&M's?

When it come to normal eating, knowing why we eat can be as important as what we eat, say experts. We can eat for the right reasons. Physical hunger, for example, when the body is depleted of fuel and needs nourishment. Food provides vital energy to power us through long busy days. We can eat for the wrong reasons, too, like when we use food to soothe emotional ups and downs; or when we are fearful of not having a full tummy.

In the midst of all that life throws our way, we can ask ourselves two questions: How am I feeling? What do I need? If I am feeling hungry, I need to eat. Bored? I need to take a walk. Tired? I need to rest. Food does its best job on physical hunger.

Sometimes we eat when we are relieved, such as when I happily munched my apple after learning my connecting flight was not cancelled after all; it was just delayed.

Sometimes we eat for comfort and because some food brings us back to our roots. Safely landed in New Mexico, my mom and daughter picked me up at the airport. And we headed straight to Cervantes' restaurant where I finally got my long-anticipated green chile fix. In the familiar surroundings with people I loved, I quickly forgot the cares of the day. And all was right with the world.

STRESS AFFECTS NUTRITION

I was trying not to feel stressed as the traffic backed up and then stopped. I was, after all, on my way to a seminar entitled, "Stress, Anxiety and Depression." I took a deep breath, which was later confirmed as a great stress reliever, and was thankful I had allowed extra time to get to my destination.

Stress affects several areas of the brain, I soon learned. For example, ever wonder why we know it's not a good idea to eat a half gallon of ice cream when we're feeling tense...but we do it anyway? Turns out the prefrontal cortex, the part of the brain that helps us make reasonable decisions, shuts down when we are stressed. Chronic stress can also alter hormones controlled by the hypothalamus, the brain's master control area; this affects appetite control and even the rate at which our bodies burn calories.

Stress is not always bad, say experts. We need some stress to survive in this world. If I'm trapped in a burning building, for example, stress hormones rapidly pump fat and sugar into my blood to help me run to safety. But when this same stress response is repeatedly turned on, whether I face a real threat or not, my blood pressure, blood sugar, and blood cholesterol remain elevated and impact my physical as well as emotional health. No wonder chronic stress is now recognized as a trigger for heart disease, cancer, stroke, lung disease, diabetes, accidents, pneumonia and flu.

When stress hormones are controlled, we sleep better while our bodies undergo repair and restore us to sanity...literally. Calm bodies digest food more efficiently and maintain more normal blood pressure, cholesterol and blood sugar levels. We can help this process happen when we embrace these habits:

- Schedule time to sleep well. Stress hormones are turned off when we are in deep sleep; this is the time that the body and brain are in restoration mode.
- Cut out caffeine at least 6 hours before beddy-bye. That's how long it takes for this stimulant to be cleared out of the body for better sleep.
- Put a lid on the bottle. Alcohol interferes with REM sleep, the deep, dream-related sleep that refreshes the brain and stores memory.
- Don't rely on sleep supplements. Products like melatonin to induce sleep only encourage our brains to make less of this natural substance, increasing the problem over time. Take sleep aids only when needed for a short term to restore natural circadian rhythm, say experts.
- Rest and digest. When we take time to calm down and eat pleasant unhurried meals, the body sends out signals that improve digestion and help keep our blood sugar levels on an even keel.
- Take time to be active. Inactivity can trigger anxiety, while regular exercise calms the stress response.
- Pick your battles. People who only stress over things they can control tend to be the healthiest and longest-lived, say experts. Which is why, as I watched the traffic back up on my drive home this day, my first thought was for ice cream. But my second thought, after I took a deep breath, was to remember the serenity prayer: "God grant me the serenity to accept the things I cannot change, courage to change the things I can, and wisdom to know the difference."

REFLECTION: An elevation in the stress hormone, cortisol, is now regarded as a reliable indicator of psychological stress. And this response helps explain why some dieters relapse to old eating habits and regain weight when they encounter stressful situations, according to experts.

Magnesium is one nutrition supplement that may help induce sound sleep, say researchers. It works on neurotransmitters in the brain that regulate sleep. For mild cases of insomnia, a dose of 400 to 800 milligrams of magnesium have been found to help the brain and muscles relax and increase the time spent in restful sleep. Best absorbed forms of magnesium include aspartate, citrate, lactate, and chloride, according the Food and Drug Administration.

COMFORTING FOOD

Some visits home are harder than others. This one was to say goodbye to my mom until I see her in heaven one day. Times of grief and loss disrupt normal routines. My sisters and I slept less. We skipped meals. We drank more coffee. Nutritional concerns flew out the window as other matters took precedence over grocery shopping and meal planning. Fortunately, we were blessed with family and friends who jumped into our lives to nourish us in more ways than we could count.

Food can indeed bring comfort in difficult times. My sisters and I, dazed from the loss of our mother, were thankful for the freshly baked cookies and hot coffee offered to us as we sat down to make plans for her funeral service. And friends and family took care of us when we weren't particularly thinking about taking care of ourselves. This was the time, we learned, to allow others to do that.

Eileen, my mom's dear friend for more than 50 years, showed up one day with a roasted chicken, fresh fruit salad, and pastries.

Bill and Adele brought essentials that we certainly needed as extended family began to gather: breakfast muffins, a huge container of ground coffee, paper plates, cups, napkins, plastic ware...and toilet paper. Mom's closest friend, Joan, arranged for a tray of meat, cheese, and freshly baked bread to be delivered to the house just as our uncle and cousins arrived from Ohio. Cousins Jan and Joan sent a basket of fresh fruit, nuts, cheese, and crackers.

Friends brought trays of cut up vegetables, homemade lasagna and green chile enchiladas. Neighbors dropped off cards and money to help with incidental expenses. On the day of Mom's service, women from her church group showed up with every conceivable type of covered dish; and they stayed to serve and feed every hungry soul that afternoon. Maryanne, Mom's neighbor we are sure is an angel, was there continually, to serve food, clean dishes, and help us get through.

The night before our uncle and cousins headed back to Ohio, we enjoyed a last meal together at a favorite New Mexican restaurant. As we ate the familiar fare, we laughed and told stories about our family. And before heading back to the reality of life, we shared one more basket of sopapillas. Looking back, my sisters and I saw how each act of kindness, from food to hugs, brought much-needed comfort. We were grateful.

WHEN FRIENDS COME TO VISIT

My best friend from eighth grade came for a visit last week; first time we've seen each other in more than 20 years. She's a teacher. I'm a nutritionist. But while she was here, we acted like we were still teenagers.

Maybe it's because Terry and I went through our adolescent growth spurts together. Those were the days when we would eat all the cookie dough before we ever baked the cookies. We could polish off a carton of ice cream with two small spoons. These days, our bodies don't burn ice cream calories quite as easily; and we're

Quinn-Essential Nutrition

more aware of our health needs. For example, a recent report on women's health and nutrition did not specifically address how many calories Terry and I burned during four days of non-stop talking. But it does warn us about extremes of body weight and osteoporosis, a condition of weakened, porous bones. Both these conditions are approaching epidemic proportions in women, according to this report.

We should have read this before we gave way to donuts and coffee on Terry's first morning here. She helped me with a garage sale, you see, and it was cold and the donuts were...there. And the next day, we weren't exactly looking for bone-building calcium-rich foods at the potluck we attended. We did stop talking long enough to enjoy several main dishes and salads, however. And then we eyed Marge's famous apple pie and something really gooey with chocolate...

This report goes on to say that more women die of heart disease and stroke than all cancers combined; and nutrition is a critical component to reduce our risk for these diseases. Thank heaven my husband threw us a few balanced-meal life preservers during Terry's visit. One evening while we talked, he served us fresh salmon with grilled vegetables. And we did manage to eat salad or fruit with most of our meals.

We even walked into town one day. And we met football icon John Madden at Bruno's Market after my dog tried to eat his barbecue sandwich. When I suggested I'd like to interview him about his cookbook, "John Madden's Ultimate Tailgating," he declined. "You won't like anything I eat," he said.

Terry smirked. "Don't kid yourself. I've known her since 8th grade. She'll eat anything."

The next day as we shared a chocolate ice cream dessert at the Big Sur River Inn, my dear friend and I realized there is no truth to the theory that calories get cancelled out when you are on vacation. So we decided to take a walk on the beach which is good for the bones. And we continued to talk about the last 20 years of our lives which is good for the soul.

Barbara A. Quinn, MS, RD, CDE

"Honestly," Terry confessed as we shared a "Bucket of Trash" at Bubba Gump Shrimp Company her last day here, "I don't always eat like this!" That's OK, Terry, neither do I.

EMOTIONAL EATING

I watched my horse eat while I cleaned out his corral. Even though he had a pile of hay right in front of him, he was poking his head between the fence railing, trying to eat his brother's hay in the next corral.

Poor Cal, since his surgery a few weeks ago, he's having a difficult time settling into recovery mode. He doesn't like being penned up. He's bored. I've noticed a change in his personality during this time of forced inactivity. He's not happy. He paws the ground. And he wants to eat, just to have something to do.

Horses aren't the only ones who turn to food to cope with stress and pain. Researcher Mary Dallman from the University of California-San Francisco found that stressed-out rats release stress-related hormones and seek out lard and sugar which she called "rat comfort food." We humans tend to do the same when we feel stressed, which may be one reason for our exploding national waistlines.

Fortunately, Cal is not allowed to eat freely from the haystack anytime he pleases. So even though his activity has been severely limited, his weight has remained stable (pardon the pun). Another reason that Cal has not ballooned into a draft horse is that he fidgets. Researchers call this "spontaneous physical activity" which, depending on the individual, accounts for 10 to 15 percent of the calories we burn each day. And we all expend this energy at different rates. While Cal paws the ground and kicks at the dog, his mother, Polly, stands quietly and stares at trees. She has much less spontaneous physical activity than her rambunctious son.

Cal tends to be calmer and not apt to get into a feeding frenzy when he knows I will feed him at regular times. With humans, too, balanced regular meals help keep appetites from going berserk. Feeling satisfied after eating is tied to hormones in the gut that turn off our urge to eat. One hormone called PPY goes into action after a high fiber meal; and Cal's hay is indeed high in fiber.

Can we increase these appetite-suppressing hormones in our body by eating certain types of food? According to Dr. Stephen Bloom, who spoke on this topic at the Scientific Sessions of the *American Diabetes Association*, the best stimulus for appetite control is a *combination* of foods that provide fat, protein, and carbohydrates. In other words, eating balanced meals may be the best medicine for controlling out of control appetites.

Cal looks forward to his daily walks, but as per doctor's orders, they cannot be too strenuous. But even our short strolls down the road and back helps keep his muscles from losing strength. Moving his body also helps burn off some of his nervous energy and makes him less grouchy. I also noticed that his walks distract him from wanting to eat all the time.

Still, Cal misses exploring trails on our usual long rides. But he will soon see that these days of confinement were temporary. One day he will be well enough to run and buck again. Until then he is learning that the grass is not always greener in his neighbor's feed bin.

CHOCOLATE: FOOD OR DRUG?

It started innocently enough; just a few sweets shared among co-workers. What could it hurt? I thought as I opened a package of M&M's given to me by a friend. After all, chocolate is a natural plant food from the seeds of the cacao tree. Cocoa butter, like all vegetable fats, contains no cholesterol. And chocolate contains stearic acid, a unique type of saturated fat that does not raise blood cholesterol levels like other types of saturated fat.

Still, I had to admit, stearic acid is only one of several types of saturated fat in chocolate. Others react as we would expect; they increase blood cholesterol levels. And even though dark chocolate generally contains less fat and sugar than milk chocolate, my chocolate goodie contains about 2 teaspoons of fat per ounce.

Barbara A. Quinn, MS, RD, CDE

But don't forget, I reminded myself as I nibbled on a chocolate chip cookie the next day, chocolate contains several antioxidant-like substances which may protect against cancer and heart disease. Nutritionally, chocolate is a significant source of magnesium which the body tends to use more during times of stress. Magnesium has been found in some studies to ease the symptoms—and the chocolate cravings—associated with premenstrual syndrome.

Later that day, at a potluck dinner, I piled my plate with salad and vegetables. But then I saw the brownies...the brownies. I don't need them, I told myself. I can walk away at any time. Deep down however, I knew these cravings were beyond what I feel for broccoli.

A review published in the *Journal of the Academy of Nutrition and Dietetics* states that chocolate may be "the most commonly craved food in North America, especially among 16 to 19 year-olds and women between 40 to 49 years of age." Chocolate, according to neuroscientists, contains several substances with drug-like actions. One is phenylethylamine which is structurally similar to amphetamine, a stimulant that transmits messages of well-being to the brain and may ease the symptoms of depression. Chocolate also contains caffeine and theobromine, substances that produce feelings sometimes described as "internal bliss."

Who can we blame? Mr. Hershey? He invented the chocolate bar in 1831. Mr. Nestle? He added sugar and dry milk to cocoa in 1875 to create milk chocolate. My mother? Scientists say we are born with a taste for sweet and fat, both which are present in chocolate.

Later, over a cup of hot chocolate, I considered my reasons to avoid eating excessive amounts of this food/drug. Chocolate can worsen heartburn by relaxing the esophageal sphincter, the "gate" that normally keeps stomach acids from sloshing up into the esophagus. But don't blame chocolate for acne. It's usually stress, say experts, not chocolate, that makes our skin erupt. For now, scientists continue to tackle this important issue. Is chocolate a food...or a drug? No ones seems to agree. I think I'll have another M&M.

TO THE HEART OF CHOCOLATE

So let's pop the question: Is chocolate good for us or not? This is what a team of researchers from the Harvard School of Public Health reported: "A growing body of evidence suggests that the consumption of foods rich in polyphenolic compounds, particularly cocoa, may have cardio-protective effects." Translation: Cocoa contains beneficial natural substances that makes our hearts happy.

One group of these helpful substances, known collectively as "flavanols," show special promise in keeping our arteries clear and flexible, say researchers. A bit of chocolate, especially the dark variety, may help lower blood pressure and keep heart disease at bay.

And there is more good news. While most saturated fat is considered "bad" because it raises the dangerous LDL cholesterol in our blood, the primary saturated fat that occurs naturally in chocolate is stearic acid, a neutral fat that does not tend to affect cholesterol levels. Recent studies have also noted that cocoa contains constituents that may help improve brain function and lower our risk for "can't remember" diseases like dementia and Alzheimers.

But alas, these truths about chocolate are bittersweet, say experts. Cocoa powder, the nonfat part of the cocoa seed that contains most of the beneficial substances, is also the most bitter-tasting. We may be wooed by sweet and creamy varieties, but they do not hold the best promise for our tender hearts.

So in chocolate as in love, it pays to look for good qualities. Chocolates richest in cocoa content also tend to be richer in heart-protective flavanols, say experts. In general, dark chocolate contains more cocoa than milk chocolate. And white chocolate contains no cocoa at all.

Thus far, there is no recommended daily dose of chocolate. Darn. However, according to Harvard researcher and epidemiologist Eric Ding, Ph.D, "We continue to uncover wide-ranging benefits of cocoa flavanols for health and longevity, and it looks like this trend will continue." I love that.

Barbara A. Quinn, MS, RD, CDE

ADVICE FROM A HORSE

It was a much needed change of pace for us all…a road trip with friends and horses to the wild blue yonder after a long winter of rain and mud. We had granola, fresh fruit and hot coffee for breakfast; then loaded up the horses and dogs and headed for the hills. On the way, we stopped at the local food market to pick up our rations—sandwiches, beverages…and a few assorted goodies.

We unloaded the horses at the top of a sweeping vista; and as he looked around, my horse, Cal, perked his ears as if to say, "Holy smokes! Where are we?"

We spent the rest of the day riding up and down the hills of this pristine valley. And my thoughts turned to a pillow that sits on the chair in my bedroom. On it, in embroidered letters, are these words of "Advice from a Horse:"

Keep the burrs from under your saddle. We can avoid major problems on the trail when Cal feels comfortable under his saddle and his load is not too heavy. I too, can avoid major health troubles if I don't pack on too much weight. Putting on the feedbag too often is now recognized as a major source of damaging inflammation in the body.

Loosen the reins. This helps Cal maneuver expected turns in the trail and keeps his head calm. Likewise, there are times when it's OK to loosen our hold on strict diet expectations. This day, we took a midday break from our long ride to devour a hearty lunch under the comforting shade of a giant white oak. It was all good.

Keep stable. Up and down the hills and valleys of our 7-mile trek, my friend Jack's mule, Henry, never missed a step. His steady pace reminded me that we make progress with consistent steps in the right direction. To lose or maintain weight, for example, we need to keep moving for 60 to 90 minutes every day, according to guidelines from the *American College of Sports Medicine* and the *American Heart Association*.

Be free-spirited. At the end of the day, we unsaddled our tired sweaty horses and turned them out into a giant green pasture. Oh, how they enjoyed the freedom to run and buck and roll!

Gallop to greatness! We were all tired, yet invigorated after this glorious day of relaxing activity. And as tired as I was, I also felt strengthened for the next big adventure!

Carry your friends when they need it. I always feel secure on the back of my strong horse, Cal. Yet it was also good to climb out of the saddle for a refreshing meal with good friends. Let's do it again soon!

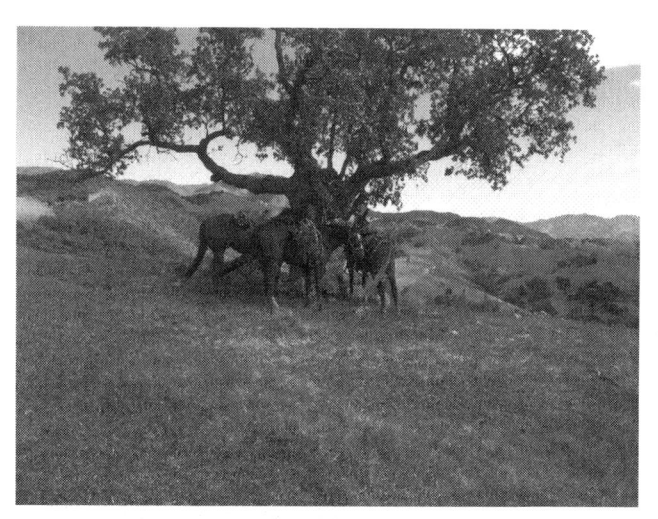

Hills above Santa Ynez, California

REFLECTION: My dear friend, Chris Regan and I continue to travel to Santa Ynez, California each year to ride in the rolling green Peach Tree hills with her dad, Jack Collison and his sure and steady mule, Henry.

FUELING ACTIVE BODIES

▓▓▓ PHYSICAL THERAPIST'S REASONS TO EXERCISE

While we sit back with super bowls of chips and dip to watch football players slug it out, we might want to think about our own health and fitness. Why? Poor eating habits and lack of physical activity are major causes of illness and death in our country. To put it simply, we eat too much of everything except vegetables and fruit. And we prefer watching people be active rather than being active ourselves.

Why is exercise so beneficial? I asked physical therapist Alain Claudel. Here are his expert reasons to be active:

- Speeds metabolism. "A well-conditioned body burns more fat by just living and breathing," Claudel explains. As muscles develop with exercise, the body requires and uses up more energy throughout the day...even when you sit to watch a football game.
- Burns calories. When we work our muscles during exercise, they become more efficient at burning calories, especially carbs and fats in such favorites as chips and cheese dip.
- Builds bones. Stress, which is the force exerted on the body when we walk or train with weights, is actually good for bones, says Claudel. These weight-bearing activities help deposit strength-building elements such as calcium, into bones.

- Improved structural integrity. "Structurally, a person who exercises is better off," he says. Like an earthquake-proof building, a strong body responds to trauma with less damage. That's why football players can withstand a hit that would land most of us in the hospital and still be able to jump up before the next commercial break.
- Lessens pain. Certain types of pain syndromes are alleviated by neural activity when nerves are stimulated, Claudel explains. "Exercise is a neural activity." And don't forget to drink plenty of water when you are active, he says. "Dehydration is what kills your muscles and tendons."
- Don't stop. "The benefits of exercise do not stop with age," Claudel says. Older people who stop being active lose the benefits quicker than when they were younger, he explains.
- Know the difference between exercise and physical activity. Both are important, he says. Exercise is repetitive, a key ingredient if you are trying to recover from an injury. Exercise has a specific purpose such as, "I'm lifting these weights so I can go out there and slam the quarterback to the ground." Physical activity means moving the body, such as taking the stairs instead of the elevator.

Exercise should not hurt, Claudel reminds us. After the game, Sunday's players may have what physical therapists call "DOMS"—delayed onset of muscle soreness. That's normal, he says. "Pain during exercise however, is *not* normal. That's when you may need to see a physical therapist."

- Challenge yourself to do something different. "If you always exercise the same muscle groups, you won't get the same benefit," he says.
- Kill your television. "It's better for us to *do* the exercise," Claudel concludes, "than to watch an immature millionaire do it."

Barbara A. Quinn, MS, RD, CDE

> REFLECTION: *According to experts at Harvard Medical School, for every two hours that we watch television each day, we increase our risk for being overweight by 25 percent. One possible reason: A study in 2012 found that the processes that manufacture fat cells are increased when our muscles are laid out and inactive for long stretches of time*

GAME PLAN FOR NUTRITION

My friend Lori has three daughters playing sports this fall, two in soccer, one in volleyball. She and her husband do their best to make it to all the games. That makes dinner, she says, "a challenge."

I remember those days with my daughters, too. I liked the soccer season best. Soccer is a timed sport; when the whistle blows, game over. And most of the soccer fields had no lights. So when the sun went down, oh darn, we had to go home and eat dinner.

Volleyball...is a different game. In those days, each event was three to five matches. And each match was played until one team scored a gazillion points. Which meant if the opposing teams had similar skills, bring your sleeping bag. What's a dedicated parent to do? Here are some tips for athletes and their faithful fans who long for dinner hour night after night:

Set some rules. Game day, no exceptions, within hours of your darling's competition, she will ingest food and/or a beverage that is easy to digest and high in carbohydrates. Examples include low fat yogurt or yogurt drinks, crackers with peanut butter, fruit juice, sports bars or beverages. Carbohydrate-containing foods, say sports nutrition experts, prep the body for competition by packing easily accessed energy into soon-to-be-active muscles.

Serve athletes fluids during competition. During intense exercise, athletes need about 8 ounces (1 cup) of fluids every 15 minutes, or 20 to 40 ounces every hour. Water is best for games lasting less than an hour (we can only hope). For longer games, add sports drinks that contain electrolytes as well as carbohydrates.

Time out. Use this brief break in the competition to stand up, wave and point for your athlete to drink some fluid.

Spike. Your athlete may be able to win the game in a hurry with this move, but only if her muscles stay fed and hydrated.

Net something reasonable from the snack bar when games go into overtime. Popcorn, pretzels, nuts, bottled water or juice can prevent faithful parents from falling off the bleachers during long games.

Point your athlete to foods with carbs (sugars and starches) within an hour or two after the game concludes. Those first 15 minutes after the stop of exercise appear to be the most critical to adequately replenish glycogen, the storage form of energy in the muscles. Easy after-the-game foods include milk, fruit or juice.

Add in a daily multi-vitamin mineral supplement if you haven't seen your athlete eat anything green since she was a baby. An age-appropriate balanced supplement contains about 100 percent of the daily value for most vitamins and minerals.

Score nutritional points by encouraging your athlete to eat adequate amounts of protein foods over the next 24 hours after a game. Meat, fish, poultry, beans, eggs, nuts and soy products contain vital amino acids that help to preserve muscle tissue, generate energy and keep your athlete's immune system strong.

Win! Face it, after-game meals aren't always nutritional winners. But at least try for three out of five.

Barbara A. Quinn, MS, RD, CDE

WRESTLING WITH MAKING WEIGHT

My friend confided that her son is trying to "make weight" for his high school wrestling team. "Last fall, he weighed 185 pounds for football," she says. "And now he's wrestling at 165. It's crazy."

It *is* crazy. In an ill-directed attempt to gain a competitive advantage by wrestling in a lower weight category, some athletes who compete under strict weight requirements will fast, restrict fluids and exercise excessively, trying to lose weight in the days or hours before a competition. What gets lost in these desperate attempts to lose weight quickly is not just fat but water and muscle. Dehydration lessens the body's ability to cool itself and makes it hard for the heart to pump blood. Less blood pumped to the muscles decreases performance and, if taken to extremes, can lead to heart and kidney damage. Maybe there's a better way. Here are some tips from sports nutrition experts:

- If you really need to lose extra body fat to compete, do it the old-fashioned way; train for it year-round. Endurance training, like running, is a good way to burn off fat. Working with weights builds muscle. But it doesn't happen overnight. Physiologically, it is next to impossible to lose more than two or three pounds of fat in a week. If you lose weight faster than that, you're probably kissing goodbye some valuable muscle mass and water.
- Stay hydrated! Remember that your muscles are 60 to 70 percent water. When you sweat off fluids to make weight, you shrink your muscular strength as well. To maintain your stamina and stay strong during training and competition, replace every pound you lose with 24 ounces of fluids.
- Eat three to four small meals during your days of training. And do not skip breakfast! This will provide a steady supply of fuel to build strength into your working muscles. Small, frequent meals can also help control your appetite so you will not be as apt to binge.

Quinn-Essential Nutrition

- Eat adequate amounts of carbohydrates (sugars and starches) and moderate amounts of protein. You need both. An athlete who avoids carbohydrates is like a hummingbird that avoids nectar. Brain and muscle cells can be easily drained of energy during intense competition without essential fuel from carbohydrate foods like fruit, grains, vegetables, milk, yogurt, pasta and beans. Carbs also help "spare" protein so this valuable nutrient isn't burned for energy but can be used for building and repairing muscle tissue.
- Choose foods that are low in fat to cut back on excess calories and lose unwanted weight. You know the drill: fruits, vegetables, baked, grilled, or roasted meat, fish or poultry, low-fat milk, yogurt and cheese.
- Stay hydrated. Yes, it's important enough to repeat. If your muscles dry up (literally) so will your competitive edge. Drink fluids before, during and after workouts. How do you know if you are well hydrated? Check the color of your urine. If it is darker than pale yellow, keep drinking. Sports nutrition experts recommend you drink 2 cups of fluid two hours before you compete. During long practices that last over an hour, drink a cup of fluid every 30 minutes. Competitions that last longer than an hour merit sports drinks that contain carbohydrates.

TOUCHDOWN: FOOTBALL NUTRITION

OK guys, listen up. I'm not your coach and I'm not your mother. But if you want to finish the season with no serious nutritional infractions, you'll need to pass this basic quiz:

1. If you sweat a lot and/or get cramps after long workouts, you may need a) a new deodorant; b) sports drinks that contain electrolytes; c) a little more salt in your diet. Answers: b and c. Muscle spasms can happen if sodium and potassium lost in sweat are not replaced.

2. Explosive energy to throw a pass or run a touchdown comes from a) your mom screaming from the stands; b) instant carbohydrate fuel in your muscles called glycogen; c) double bacon cheeseburgers. Answer: b. Glycogen supplied by carbohydrate-rich foods is an immediate source of energy for working muscles. High fat foods (like cheeseburgers) take longer to digest and can s-l-o-w you d-o-w-n.
3. Day after day of football drills can a) deplete your muscles of glycogen; b) make you wish you were a cowboy; c) increase your need for high carbohydrate foods. Answers: a and c. Muscles rebuild their energy stores when supplied with carbs and scheduled rest.
4. Some healthful examples of high carb foods are a) bagels; b) beans; c) fruit; d) yogurt. Answer: All are correct.
5. The most frequently overlooked aid to enhance your athletic performance is a) roughing the passer; b) proper hydration; c) popping a 60-yard field goal. Answer: b. Muscles perform better and longer when they contain adequate amounts of fluid.
6. You may not be getting enough fluids if a) you feel dizzy or light-headed; b) your urine is dark in color; c) you get sick to your stomach during practice. Answer: All of these can be signs of dehydration.
7. True or False? During intense activity, your body generates 15 to 20 times more heat than usual. Answer: True.
8. Failure to drink enough fluid in extreme hot or cold weather can cause a) unsportsmanlike conduct; b) heatstroke; c) poor athletic performance. Answers: b and c
9. Athletes need to consume water a) one or two hours *before* practices and games; b) every 15 to 20 minutes *during* practices and games; c) *after* every practice and game. Answer: YES! ALL of these are appropriate times to refill your fluid stores.
10. It's important to sip fluids before you feel thirsty because a) exercise can throw your thirst signals out of whack;

Quinn-Essential Nutrition

b) dehydration is for sissies; c) water bottles are cool. Answer: a
11. For practices or games lasting less than one hour, the best fluid to drink is a) non-alcoholic beer; b) plain water; c) sweet tea. Answer: b.
12. If your practice or game lasts *more* than one hour, you may need a) extra players; b) sports drinks that contain carbohydrates and electrolytes; c) a winning season. Answer: b.

OWNERS MANUAL FOR THE HUMAN MACHINE

Note: This column coincided with the prestigious Pebble Beach Concours d'Elegance, one of the top-ranking car competitions in the world. On the third week of August each year, international car enthusiasts converge on the Monterey Peninsula for a grand show and sale of rare and very expensive automobiles.

Expect to see some pretty elegant cars around town this week. And some very meticulous owners who bestow extensive care on these high quality vehicles. Our human bodies are high caliber vehicles as well; and they'll carry us in style if we give them good care. Still, the journey can be long and the roads can get bumpy. Some parts will need to be fixed along the way, and a few can be replaced. If an instruction manual came with your body, here is what it might include:

Fuel requirements will vary, depending on the age and condition of your vehicle. Human engines derive energy, or calories from four sources: carbohydrates (sugars and starches), protein, fat, and alcohol. Complete combustion of one gram of protein, sugar or starch produces four calories of energy; fat produces twice this amount, or nine calories. Whatever the source, adult engines used for daily driving usually require about 12 to 15 calories of fuel per pound of chassis weight.

Barbara A. Quinn, MS, RD, CDE

Use high quality fuel. Breakdowns may occur with less than optimal energy sources. Carbohydrates derived from whole grains, fruit, vegetables and low fat milk or yogurt have been found to provide the cleanest, most efficient fuel for human engines. Fuel efficiency is further enhanced with additives that contain B-vitamins such as enriched or whole grain breads or cereals, nuts and legumes.

Refuel regularly. For top efficiency, your human vehicle requires fuel at the beginning of each daily journey. Stop to refuel about every 4 to 6 hours until you park your engine for the night. Headache and sluggish uphill climbs may signal poor fuel economy. If you get a warning light that you are low on fuel, pull over and do not attempt to operate your vehicle until you correct the problem.

Control emissions. Frequent backfiring may indicate a problem in your emission control system. Check the fiber content on the Nutrition Facts panel when you purchase high-efficiency carbohydrate fuels. Superior additives are whole grains, nuts, and beans that contain at least 8 to 10 percent Daily Value for dietary fiber.

Correct fluid leaks immediately. Top performance human engines require a liter of clean water for every 1000 calories of fuel burned. Caution: Engine parts may be damaged if fluid is not added on a regular basis, especially in hot weather or when climbing mountain grades.

If your vehicle stalls, do not attempt to push or tow it to restart the engine. Head for the nearest overnight rest stop and allow your built-in catalytic energy converter to regenerate. Check gauges the following morning and refuel as necessary.

Do not allow your engine to idle at high speeds. Damage to internal parts may result. Blow our excess steam and carbon with daily exercise and deep breathing.

Quinn-Essential Nutrition

Do not overload your vehicle's carrying capacity. Refer to your owner's manual for recommended load limits.

Engine additives may be beneficial in some circumstances. Antique vehicles over the age of 50 for example, may require extra vitamin B-12 from fortified foods and supplements to assure adequate fuel efficiency, according to experts. Check with your trained human maintenance professional to further evaluate requirements for your specific model.

GOLF TERMS

Just in case Kevin Costner is looking for me at the AT&T Pebble Beach Pro-Am, I'll be with the other volunteers at the food tent run by a guy we affectionately call "Nick the Slavedriver."

The work is quite fun. Sometimes we get to put tomatoes and pickles on hamburger buns. Other times we get to serve beer to stoked tournament attendees. And sometimes Nick even lets us take a break. I seem to know more about a chicken sandwich than a birdie. But during my time as a food tent volunteer, I have learned these common golf terms:

Tee. Both green and black teas contain substances called "flavonoids" that have proven health benefits. Flavonoids in black tea exert protection against heart disease while those in green tea help defend the body from certain types of cancer.

Fore! What a great way to remind us that we need to eat four servings of vegetables (about 2 cups) every day. And I believe the rule is to yell this out as soon you meet this daily quota.

Iron. It's an important tool for golf as well as nutrition. Iron is a carrier of life-saving oxygen that drives energy. Tannins in foods such as tea can block the absorption of iron, so best not to tea off at the same time.

Barbara A. Quinn, MS, RD, CDE

Hole in one. I assume golfers use this term to describe bagels or doughnuts. They seem to be quite fond of them.

Stroke. Golfers must strive to have these less often. Medically, our risk for having a "heart attack in the brain" goes up if we drink too much alcohol, eat too much fat, and consume too few vegetables and whole grains.

Par 15. I believe this golf term denotes the dollar amount of what you'll pay for a chicken sandwich, chips, and beverage at our food tent this weekend.

Greens. Expect to see more of these on the course than in our food tent.

Putt. This action during the tournament requires all spectators to chew their burgers quietly.

Hazard. You may experience this if you yell and wave at Kevin Costner while he is concentrating on his tin cup.

Water. It surrounds some of the world's most beautiful golf courses. It carries nourishment and energy to our bodies. And we've got that for you in our food tent.

EAT, SLEEP SWIM: WHAT CHAMPIONS DO

I jotted down American swimmer Michael Phelps' answer when he was asked what he would do after winning his first gold medal of the 2008 Beijing Olympics. "Eat, sleep, and swim." he said.

Good answer; and it must be working. At the time of this writing, Phelps was on his way to breaking several Olympic records. According to one report, Phelps ate about 12,000 calories a day while training for competition; that's a *lot* of calories. In comparison, an average American eats about 2000 calories a day and doesn't look near as good in swim trunks.

What does Phelps eat? "A lot of pizza and pasta," he told one reporter. "I'm eating carbs (sugars and starches) and sleeping as much as I can." Top athletes know the best way to come back day after day to win medal after medal is not to let their muscles get fatigued. Carbohydrate-rich foods combined with adequate rest after workouts restore high octane fuel to tired muscles. Higher amounts of this fuel, or glycogen, packed into muscles increase an athlete's advantage to keep going strong in competition.

"Carbohydrates are the main fuel for high intensity exercise," writes sports science professor Clyde Williams and exercise physiology professor David Lamb. "The more demanding the training program or competition, the greater is the amount of dietary carbohydrate needed to replace glycogen stores. Failure to replace muscle stores of glycogen results in the inability to maintain an optimum race pace during endurance competitions."

Of course protein and fat are also important for athletes. In addition to carbs, fat is a valuable fuel for working muscles. Protein is essential to build and repair weary muscles. In addition, protein delivers essential nutrients and oxygen to the energy-producing cells of a hard-working body.

But don't try the 12,000-calorie pizza and pasta diet at home, boys and girls. Not unless you are ready to jump into the pool and swim and swim and swim along with other types of intense exercise. To stay in good shape, we can eat more calories only if we *burn* more calories through physical activity.

Athletes with rippling muscles have another advantage than just looking good in Speedos. Muscles are the body's metabolically active tissue. That means people with more muscles burn more calories for fuel, even when they are sleeping. And because athletes burn more calories, they can eat more calories without becoming fat.

Barbara A. Quinn, MS, RD, CDE

REFLECTION: Michael Phelps won eight gold medals in the 2008 Beijing Olympics. In 2012, he won four golds and two silver medals in the Summer Olympics in London, making him the most decorated Olympian of all time.

RACE REGIMEN

I indirectly experimented with carbohydrate loading many years ago; the athlete was my horse. I was (kind of) working on my Uncle Don's ranch in Meeker, Colorado one summer when a friend persuaded me to enter my mare, Nicky, in a local horse race. He had seen her speed and knew that she had been a race horse before I bought her. He agreed to ride her in the race and I agreed to get her ready for the competition.

I soon learned that my uncle had entered his best horse in this race; and like many of the other ranchers, he had a sizable chunk of money riding on his steed.

So Nicky and I started her training schedule. She got frequent workouts around the track and plenty of fresh water. Twice a day, I gave her high quality hay with supplements of oats, corn, and molasses. As race day drew near, I gradually fed her less high fiber hay and more high carb grain.

My uncle didn't pay much attention. He didn't see the need to increase his horse's exercise routine or change his hay-centered diet. Need I mention who was standing in the winner's circle at the end the race? And whose horse came in dead last...with a tummy full of undigested hay? Suffice it to say, my uncle was not terribly amused by the good fortune of his hired hand.

Sports athletes know that the right training combined with adequate hydration and a high octane diet can greatly influence the results of competition. Here are some tips:

Training: The best fuel for working muscles comes from carbohydrates which are the sugars and starches found in fruit, grains, vegetables, milk and yogurt. However, muscles can only store a limited amount of carbohydrates, or glycogen. So these glycogen stores become the limiting factor that determines how long you can exercise, says sports nutrition expert Nancy Clark. Endurance athletes who train for events that last longer than 90 minutes should carb load *every* day, says Clark. That requires them to eat about 60 to 70 percent of their total calories from carbohydrate foods. It's been shown that this eating style combined with a focused training program can actually stimulate muscles to store more energy. On race day, that translates to increased stamina and go power.

And hear this, you weekend runners: packing in the pasta the night before a race won't necessarily peak out the glycogen in your muscles *unless* you have also trained adequately for your event. It's the combination of exercise and a high carbohydrate intake over time that most benefits the energy storing capacity of muscles.

Training days are also the best times to assess your body's need for fluids, says Clark. She advises athletes to weigh themselves before and after workouts and replace two cups (16 ounces) of fluid for every pound they lose. And use training days to practice drinking different types of fluids, she advises. Learn which fluids you tolerate best, so you don't have any surprises on race day.

Traditionally, carbohydrate loading starts the week before a competition. This is when muscles can be tricked to store more glycogen and extend the time before a competitor "hits the wall." One technique, proposed by sports physiologists, starts with the athlete doing an intense workout.

Over the next five days, the competitor cuts back on the length of workouts while gradually decreasing carbohydrate intake. Three days before competition, the athlete trains and resumes his or her high carb diet. About 24 hours before the competition, the athlete rests (does not train) to allow the muscles to load up with glycogen energy.

Be careful, however. Sports nutritionist Ellen Coleman cautions against intense carbohydrate loading, especially if you have a medical condition such as diabetes or high blood triglyceride levels.

Race day. By this time, top athletes are walking storehouses of muscle fuel. To maintain these energy stores, experts say to eat a meal that is high in carbohydrates, low in fat and readily digested (no trucker's breakfasts, please) within two to three hours before competition.

It's important for athletes to maintain adequate intakes of fluids before and during competition as well. Seasoned runners know from experience how they can stay well hydrated before a race. Race day is not the day to experiment. It is not unusual for marathoners to lose two to four liters (8 to 16 cups!) of sweat during a marathon, say experts. Physician and past marathoner, Dr. Gary Grant, says the average runner competing in moderate weather conditions needs about a cup of water or balanced electrolyte solution every half hour. And don't just rely on plain water, experts warn. Electrolyte solutions and fruit replace important nutrients that keep the body functioning at its peak. Solutions that contain sodium and chloride (salt) are also important for athletes who lose large volumes of sweat during exercise.

Post exercise. One to two hours after a race is when muscles are most receptive to replacing depleted glycogen energy stores. This is a good time to consume fruit, juice, bread or other carbohydrate-rich foods and beverages. After you have pranced around the winner's circle, that is.

REFLECTION: Strategies to load carbohydrates into muscle for enhanced endurance continue to be supported by sports nutrition experts. Certified sports nutritionist and marathon runner Stephanie Bouquet also emphasizes that athletes need to carb load daily, not just the night before a race, to make sure glycogen stores are filled.

Quinn-Essential Nutrition

"Carbs fuel the muscle and brain," she adds, "but protein is the oil that keeps the motor running; so it's a good accompaniment to a carb-based meal. As part of your training regimen, have a small amount of protein at each meal. Endurance athletes have higher protein needs than the general population but not as much as everyone thinks. Most endurance athletes need about 0.6 grams of protein for every pound of body weight or 1.2 - 1.4 grams per kilogram."

Bouquet also stresses the importance of refueling as you run your race. If you don't, your body will slow down and your performance will suffer.

EATING ON THE ROAD

ROAD TRIP NUTRITION

Our family likes to take road trips, usually to visit family in New Mexico or Colorado. Why we think this is fun, no one knows. Here are some lessons learned on a road trip through the desert Southwest and cool Rocky Mountains.

- You can get your kicks on Route 66, but you'll have to look closely for vegetables. Green and red usually indicate nutritionally superior foods. New Mexico green chile and fresh tomatoes from Colorado are two good examples. Exceptions include Arizona cactus candy and anything in Needles.
- While careening down the interstate thinking about your next stop, remember that you can only justify the trucker's breakfast if you load and unload the truck.
- Learn healthful travel habits from your dog. Run around and have some fresh water at each rest stop. And take only small nibbles of food until you get to your destination.
- Best bets for snacks: oranges that can be easily peeled on cruise control. Worst bets for fruit: peaches in a bag the dog sat on, or anything from the Petrified Forest.
- Potato chips can only be counted as nourishment when your kids have eaten everything else in the car and your husband won't stop for lunch. If he finally stops for dinner after you ate all the potato chips, a salad bar is a good idea.

Quinn-Essential Nutrition

- Trail mix offers a convenient balance of nutrients for travel. Dried fruit and nuts provide a good combination of quick and long-lasting energy, and more fiber than the cream pie your husband bought in Pagosa Springs.
- Sandwiches taste better when you remember not to pack them under two bottles of water. And lastly, just because a man dressed like a taco waves at you from a fast food restaurant in Gallup, you don't have to stop.

MINNESOTA NICE

My daughter was there to present research at a conference. I was there to act like I wasn't her mother when she talked to big wigs. And we were both there to explore Minneapolis for the first time.

Nice city and very nice people, I remarked to a young man on my flight back home. "Minnesota nice," he said matter-of-factly. "You haven't heard that before?" Can't say I had. But apparently Minnesota's mostly German and Norwegian population has a reputation for being nice. (Note: We were visiting in July, not January.)

Minnesota's state beverage is milk. Their official state grain is wild rice. Locals put these together with carrots and other vegetables to make their renowned Wild Rice Soup, which was very nice.

Surprisingly, the state bird in this "Land of 10,000 Lakes" is *not* the mosquito. It is the common loon. And if you are looking for a nice hot dish in Minnesota, be aware this is another word for casserole.

Two notable nutrition discoveries came out of the great state of Minnesota. K-rations were simple yet nutritious meals developed at the University of Minnesota for combat soldiers during World War II. This institution is also the birthplace of the Mediterranean Diet.

In 1967, Dr. Ansel Keys from the University of Minnesota's School of Public Health, began to investigate the lifestyle habits of men in the United States, Japan, Greece, Italy and Finland and their risk for heart disease. On the Greek island of Crete, his team

Barbara A. Quinn, MS, RD, CDE

observed significantly fewer cases of heart disease compared to men in the United States and Finland.

Most of these Greek men were full-time farmers who were "poor but not lacking in food," Keys noted. They ate what they grew; vegetables, lentils, grains, olives and olive oil provided the bulk of their diets. Fish, meat and dairy foods were available in small amounts. This pattern of eating which Keys described as "nutritionally good but not luxurious" became known as the "Mediterranean Diet."

Keys apparently lived what he learned. One source reported that he "generally shunned food fads and vigorously promoted the benefits of reasonably low fat diets instead of following the North American habit for making the stomach the garbage disposal unit for a long list of harmful foods." Keys died just two months short of his 101st birthday in 2002. I'm sure he was a very nice man.

REFLECTION: Like the 10,000 lakes in Minnesota, there are several versions of the Mediterranean diet. Still, the eating styles of many people in Mediterranean countries are similar. Fruit, vegetables, whole grains, beans, nuts, legumes, and olive oil are standard fare. Fish is frequently on the menu along with moderate amounts of poultry, eggs, cheese and yogurt. Desserts and red meat are eaten less often. Because of its observed health benefits, many experts, including the Harvard School of Public Health, consider the Mediterranean diet to be superior to other patterns of eating.

NEBRASKA RED

The airlines were under red alert as we traveled out of California to attend our daughter's commencement ceremony. It was just the beginning of a week of "red" in the great state of Nebraska.

Quinn-Essential Nutrition

We checked into our hotel in downtown Lincoln and the nice young man at the front desk described the special amenities of our particular room. "You have a refrigerator, microwave, and a north-facing window with a preferred view," he said proudly.

Preferred view? As soon as we got to our room, we pulled back the curtains. Sure enough, there it was—a perfect view of Memorial Stadium, home to the University of Nebraska Cornhuskers "Big Red" football team.

Red runs deep in Nebraska. It's the dress code for "Husker gear" that everyone in the state wears to football games, restaurants, and graduation ceremonies.

Red beer is a Nebraska original, I was told. A mixture of tomato juice and beer, it appears to be a routine way to supplement the Nebraskan diet with lycopene, the red antioxidant in tomatoes that protects against heart disease and certain types of cancer.

Red meat was definitely on the menu at the Lincoln Rib Fest, an outdoor barbecue event that featured champion rib grillers from as far away as Australia, Tennessee, and even Texas. Beef, pork and lamb are red because they contain more iron-containing proteins called myoglobin and hemoglobin than poultry and fish. Myoglobin stores oxygen; hemoglobin transports oxygen. Interestingly, the leaner cuts of meat are "redder" than fattier cuts. That's because lean cuts are from muscles that get more exercise and thus require more oxygen, and thus more myoglobin.

No one at this rib fest asked me, but four to six ounces of meat (about the size of a farmer's hand) is considered the most healthful way to include red meat in the diet. And while beef can be a significant source of saturated fat—the fat associated with an increased risk for heart disease—it also contains a healthful fat called conjugated linoleic acid (CLA). This fatty acid is currently under study for its potential to reduce risks for cancer and heart disease.

My eyes turned misty red the next day as we watched our daughter march into the arena in her red cap and gown to complete her college career. And my face was red hot that evening after a few aerobic rounds of Nebraska-style country western dancing.

Barbara A. Quinn, MS, RD, CDE

HOLIDAY TRAVEL DIET

This unique nine-day diet is designed for people in reasonably good health who travel long distances (such as across four western states) to visit family and friends for the holidays. Nutritional adequacy is not guaranteed. Weight results may vary.

Day 1: Get up at 5 a.m. and drive 100 miles. Stop for gas and convince yourself you need a cup of hot coffee and an apple fritter from that bakery you just drove past. Drive another 300 miles or until you are hungry again, whichever comes first. Go directly past the golden arches and take a chance that you may find something better at a place called "Chinese Food/Donut Shop." Arrive at your in-laws' house later that evening and accept their kind offer to go out to dinner. Order a salad.

Day 2: Enjoy a healthful breakfast of fresh fruit, whole grain cereal and low fat milk with your relatives before heading out on the next lap of your trip. Drive for a few hours and stop for gas. Become overwhelmed by the smell of fresh popcorn that becomes your lunch. Arrive at your destination to take your daughter and her friends out to their favorite dinner spot that features "Road Kill Burger."

Day 3: Wake up and pull an orange out of your bag. Eat one. Check out of your hotel and consciously walk past the donuts and sausage at the all-you-can-eat breakfast bar. Pour a cup of coffee and have some hot oatmeal and raisins.

Day 4: Drive to the nearest Starbucks; order a gingerbread latte and a bran muffin…because you need it. Drive as fast as the speed limit allows until you reach New Mexico. Stop at the first cafe that serves green chile. Finish your meal and take a few bites of your daughter's chicken enchiladas while she is in the ladies' room.

Day 5: Arrive at your mom's house and the next morning, drink approximately one gallon of coffee while you visit with family members. Around 6 pm, collectively decide to go out for New Mexican green chile.

Day 6: Wake up early and chase down a multivitamin with a glass of orange juice. Spend the rest of the day celebrating the holiday with your family. Take a walk around the block. Consider another walk around the block when your cousin shows up with three more pies and your son-in-law arrives with his sister's famous peanut butter fudge.

Day 7: Have a cup of coffee and a piece of leftover pie for breakfast and consider going out for a 100-mile run.

Day 8: Leave before dawn for your long drive home. Around mid-morning, pop open the giant can of popcorn your mother-in-law gave you. Around noon, replace the lid and vow to never be alone in the car with that much popcorn again. Drink two bottles of water and floss the popcorn out of your teeth, being careful to keep your eyes on the road. Find a comfortable hotel for the night and go to a real restaurant for dinner. Order a spinach salad.

Day 9: Get up early to drive the final stretch home. Do not stop at "Big Bun Boy" or be tempted by "tequila candy with genuine worm" at the truck stop. Promise you will eat nothing but fruit and vegetables for the rest of your life. Arrive home tired but safe and mostly sound. Go to bed and dream of pumpkin pie and whipped cream.

NUTRITION MILE MARKER

This year was one of those mile marker birthdays for my mom. So we thought, what the heck, let's take a little road trip from New Mexico to Nebraska and make a few stops in Colorado and Wyoming while we're at it. We started off in our all-weather (thank you, God) vehicle for a spring drive. As the miles whizzed by, we talked about years past; and I could see that mom has weathered them gracefully.

Researchers who study those who live at least 100 years find these traits in common: good genes, staying mentally and physically active, not smoking, not being obese, and being involved with family.

Our nutritional needs change as we age, however. According to a recent report by the *Academy of Nutrition and Dietetics*, a woman in her eighties needs 600 to 800 *fewer* daily calories than she did when she was twenty. Older men require 1000 to 1200 fewer calories each day than in their younger years. While our aging bodies need fewer calories, they require just as many, and sometimes more, vitamins and minerals. And for some older folks, this nutrient-dense, calorie-poor diet can be a challenge.

Adding years to our lives does have rewards, we discovered on the first evening of our excursion. To celebrate Mom's special birthday, we headed for a classy Italian restaurant in Grand Junction. As we considered the menu choices, my daughter noticed an invitation on the table that read, "Join us on your birthday and get one percent off your meal for every year of your age." Score! Let's just say the waiter got a very good tip.

As we continued on our journey, we soon realized we didn't need the truckers' breakfast unless we aspired to look like one. I followed Mom's lead to seek out hotels that offered light but nourishing morning fare such as bran muffins, fresh fruit, yogurt...and coffee.

Researchers say we eat better when we don't eat alone. And boy, was that true while visiting our other daughter in western Nebraska. As we dined with new friends around a large table at her neighbor's ranch, I watched in amazement as mom polished off her meal amidst the fun and laughter.

How we choose to eat over the mile markers of life profoundly influences our long-term health, say experts. And in spite of detours and hazardous conditions along the way, moderation and variety remain two of the most important keys to nutritional health. I learned those lessons from my mom a long time ago.

GIRLS IN THE CITY

Mandy, Mikey, and Bobbi were friends. One day they decided to drive to the big city to celebrate Mandy's birthday. "Let's have fun!" said Mandy.

"Yes, let's!" chimed Mikey and Bobbi.

So they drove and drove. Then Mandy said, "I'm hungry Let's find a place to eat."

"Yes, let's!" echoed Mikey and Bobbi.

Mandy drove to a little Mexican restaurant near the neighborhood where she once lived. They sat down and ordered a giant burrito the color of the Mexican flag. And they shared it because they were good girls and did not want to spoil their dinner plans. Bobbi ordered a side of salmon tacos because she is a dietitian and wanted to get her daily quota of omega-3 fatty acids. Mandy and Mikey just smiled.

Then Bobbi spotted some innocent-looking slivers of jalapeno peppers that Mandy was enjoying with her burrito. "Try one!" said Mandy encouragingly. "They are very mild." So Bobbi did, thankful that these tiny peppers were loaded with fiber and vitamins A and C. And they tasted very good. So she had another, and another.

"Yikes!" yelled Bobbi. "My tongue is on fire!" Mandy and Mikey just laughed.

So the girls decided to do some sightseeing to walk off their giant burrito. They saw beautiful plants and butterflies at the Conservatory. They learned new words such as "psychophily" which refers to plants that butterflies love. And they watched multi-hued butterflies slurp nectar out of red, orange, yellow and pink flowers, the colors to which they are most attracted.

Soon the girls became restless. "Let's drive to my favorite chocolate store!" Mandy suggested.

"Yes, let's!" Mikey and Bobbi agreed.

And so they did. Each friend carefully chose one special piece of chocolate, because they were good girls and did not want to spoil their appetite for dinner. And the store clerk offered them additional free samples. And it was all very good.

And the girls had a wonderful day. They meandered through the Japanese Tea Gardens. They visited the buffalo and admired the art work in Golden Gate Park. They got stuck in traffic on the way to Coit Tower; and they got stuck in traffic driving down Lombard Street. As the sun began to set, the girls said in unison, "Let's eat dinner!"

"I know just the place," said Mandy. She drove to the Fog City Diner and ordered a special meal (and chocolate cake for dessert) to celebrate their special friend's birthday.

Darkness settled onto the city and the girls were very tired. "Who will keep me awake on the drive home?" Mandy asked.

"We will!" said Mikey and Bobbi. And so they did. And the friends agreed it was a very good day indeed.

RULES FOR FLYING

I learned two important lessons from my trip across the country. One: Always pack a carry-on bag with every fathomable thing you may need for your trip. Two: Do not lose that bag. Flying can present other challenges as well. See how you might handle these:

1. What might be a good choice for an in-flight meal when breakfast was a piece of toast and you're going to miss dinner at your destination because you forgot to figure in the time change? A. fresh salad made with chopped Romaine lettuce, roasted turkey, tomatoes, light vinaigrette dressing and beautifully pictured in the in-flight magazine; B. snack box of pita chips, hummus, cheese and piece of candy; C. free pretzels and a diet soda. Answer: Sorry, selection A is not available on this flight.
2. What should you do when you arrive at your destination at 10 p.m. and your luggage does not? A. Ask the cab driver to take you to the nearest WalMart, stat; B. Go to bed and pray your luggage shows up before your important breakfast meeting in the morning; C. Go to bed and pray breakfast is not pretzels and diet soda. Answer: All are appropriate.

Quinn-Essential Nutrition

3. What is a good choice for dinner when you arrive in New York the next evening feeling dead-tired and hungry? A. Room service; B. beef scaloppini with mushrooms and peppers at a famous restaurant across the street from your hotel. Answer: Take a guess.
4. Does the complimentary milk chocolate toffee in your hotel room count as a serving of dairy if you top it off with a calcium supplement? Nice try.
5. What is the price of room service in New York for a nutritious breakfast of granola, yogurt and fresh fruit? A. $20; B. $44; C. priceless. Answers: B and C.
6. How many cups of coffee are recommended for airline travel? Answer: One, when you arrive back at the airport after four hours of sleep because you got bumped from your flight home the night before. Two, from the apologetic flight attendant when your homebound plane gets diverted to Los Angeles for a few hours. Three, when you have to call your boss to explain that you may not be at work that day.
7. Why is tonic "water" more like soda in calories and sugar content and club "soda" is more like plain water? I have no idea.
8. What can you learn from less than pleasant travel adventures? High fiber granola bars are precious life savers when meals are missed. Carry-on luggage should always contain at least one bag of nuts. Breathe; enjoy the journey; and be very thankful when you finally arrive back home.

REFLECTION: I'm not one to snap photos of everything I eat. But I couldn't resist this Stetson Chop Salad at an eatery called Cowboy Ciao in the Phoenix Airport. A rainbow of arugula, smoked salmon, couscous, chopped tomato relish, sun-dried corn, dried currants and pumpkin seeds, tossed in a dressing of herbed buttermilk. If you see an enthusiastic server named T.J., tell him I said, Hi.

Barbara A. Quinn, MS, RD, CDE

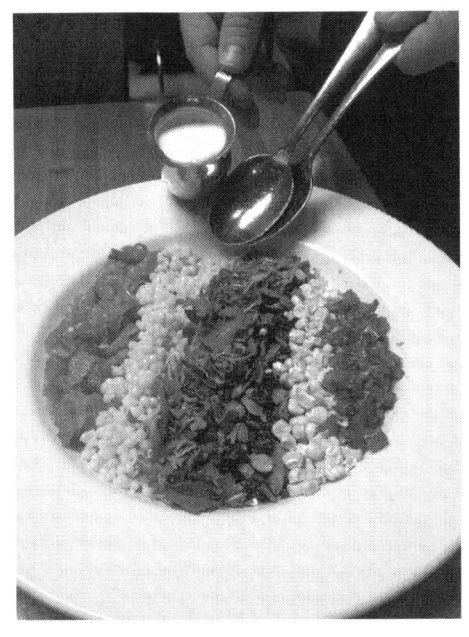

Chopped Salad at Cowboy Ciao, Phoenix Airport

FOOTBALL PORTIONS

"I get it! It's all about portions," a patient told me as we discussed a diet to control his diabetes. I heartily agree; portion control could cure a lot of what ails us in this big country of ours. Yet Americans are confused about what constitutes healthful serving sizes, I learned at a nutrition conference I attended in Philadelphia. And boy, was that driven home when another dietitian and I dined at a popular restaurant in our hotel that evening.

This steak house was owned by ex-NFL football coach, Don Shula. When we arrived, the hostess seated us and handed me a football…a real football. "It's the menu," she explained. Very cute, we said. We perused the offerings on the side of the pigskin when a waiter appeared with a cartload of main course selections.

"May I interest you ladies in our popular 48-ounce porterhouse steak? Or perhaps this 32-ounce prime rib? Or our famous 22-ounce lamb chops?" I thought he was kidding. "We get a lot of football players," he explained. "The Philadelphia Eagles were here last night."

Who really eats 48 ounces (more than two pounds) of steak at one time? I asked.

"Two hundred people so far," the waiter confidently replied. "We have a list on the wall over there."

I later learned that more than 19,000 people have joined Shula's prestigious 48-ounce club by merely downing that much steak in one sitting. For their feat, members receive a picture of Coach Shula and a personalized letter from his son, Dave. One man who ate one hundred 48-ounce steaks (not at the same time, I assume) got a free commemorative football. He was, according to Coach Shula, "a very *big* fan."

We are dietitians, I explained to the waiter. "Oh...well...then maybe you'd like seafood," he offered, holding up a five-pound Maine lobster. Or maybe this lovely one pound chicken breast."

Anything...smaller? I asked. We eventually settled on a 12-ounce filet mignon that our waiter assured us we could split. And we ordered vegetables and a glass of red wine, each.

What's the lesson here? A "portion" (the amount of food we choose to eat) is not always the same as a healthful "serving." For example, some football players may consider three pounds of meat on their plate a "portion." Registered dietitians would define that much meat as 12 "servings." Big difference, since most of us need just two or three servings of meat or other protein-rich foods each day for good health. Yep, it's all about portions. And we've got a lot to learn.

REFLECTION: As of 2015, Don Shula's 48-ounce Club boasted 39,812 beef-loving members.

SPECIAL OCCASION NUTRITION

BRIAN'S MILLENNIUM FEAST

It was a New Year's "Babette's Feast" in Portland, Oregon. That's the name of a movie that describes a once-in-a-lifetime meal lovingly prepared for guests by a very special chef.

My brother-in-law Brian's Millennium Feast was just that. He and his staff at his Ivy House Restaurant pulled out all the stops for 40 guests—Quinn's, friends, and specially invited patrons. In nutrition terms, it was the "one-in-a-thousand" rule. You'll have 999 sensible meals in your life before you get the pleasure of one like this:

First course: Northwest salmon gravlox, cured with Hood River apple brandy. Nice choice, thought my dietitian brain. Omega-3 fatty acids, fish oils found in dark-fleshed fish like salmon, are heart healthful. It was served with fresh salad greens, which provided a nice touch of fiber and folate, a B-vitamin found in "foliage."

As we dined, Brian served his 40 guests with just one bottle of champagne. Never mind that is was a 12-liter bottle with a cork big enough to blow off the roof.

Second course: Seafood bisque with rosemary baguette croutons. Yum yum!

Third course: Braised winter vegetable strudel lovingly wrapped in a flaky pastry. Good job, Brian!

Fourth course: Roasted breast of goose, thinly sliced over *Chanterelle* mushroom risotto, served with brother Steve's famous homemade 1996 Pinot Noir. And we know the benefits of red wine, do we not?

Intermission: Good idea; we took time from this five-hour meal to walk outside, breathe deeply, and think about the next four courses.

Fifth course: Cranberry sorbet with fresh mint, served with sparkling water. Light! Refreshing! And it prepared our tummies for the next round.

Sixth course: Fresh Dungeness crab, compliments of my seafaring brother-in-law, Tom.

Seventh course: Confession, this diner has basic tastes. Serve me a bit of simply prepared meat, fish or poultry, and I'm happy. On this night, however, every shred of Beef Wellington with Oregon black truffle duxelle paired with premium goose liver pate' and veal demi-glace went down this palette...along with a glass of 1982 Kenwood Cabernet Savignon.

The only way to top this meal was a proposal of marriage, which one guest popped on his unsuspecting girlfriend. Her answer? "I didn't wait eight years to say 'No'!"

Then the fireworks began...outside, I mean. Brian's pyrotechnic maniac neighbor, Phil, ushered in the new century with a light show that rivaled Paris. Energized, we sat down for the grand finale: Chocolate hazelnut torte with espresso buttercream frosting. Be still, my dietitian heart.

Toasts to the chef. Toasts to the guests. Toasts to family and friends. And nothing but toast, please, for breakfast the next morning. Mark Twain once said, "Part of the secret of success in life is to eat what you like and let the food fight it out inside." And what a fight to the finish it was. Thank you, dear Brian!

Barbara A. Quinn, MS, RD, CDE

NEW YEAR EXPECTATIONS

So you've resolved to do better this year, lose that extra weight, exercise more, get in shape. But if these same resolutions come back year after year, this may be the time to approach your goals a bit differently.

Set expectations, not resolutions. Resolving to "get more exercise this year" is a wish, not a goal. Decide instead what you specifically expect and say it out loud. "This week, I will exercise for 20 minutes over my lunch hour on Tuesday and Thursday." Don't just resolve to "eat more fruit and vegetables." Plan a strategy you expect to work into your life. One example might be, "I will add a cup of vegetables to my lunch each day this week."

Stop dieting. "Every diet has an equal and opposite binge," says registered dietitian, Lisa Holden. "Depriving yourself of food when you are truly hungry will eventually lead to overeating." Instead, Holden advises, "choose foods you enjoy and listen to your body's signals about how much to eat."

Weight management expert and registered dietitian, Michelle Barth, agrees. "The basic approach is not to go on a diet, but to find compromises in eating and exercise that you are willing to live with for the rest of your life."

Keep a food diary. Keep track of what and when you eat throughout the day. This makes eating a conscious (versus unconscious) activity, says Barth. "Your food diary helps you see very clearly what you need to change and helps track your progress."

Become more active. "Any activity is better than no activity," explains Barth. "Park farther away when you go shopping; use the stairs. Then work into some type of consistent daily activity, like walking."

Eat only when you are physically hungry. This can be tough, to eat only when your stomach feels empty and to stop eating when you no longer feel physical hunger. If you eat when you are bored or mad or sad or any other emotional reason, ask yourself these questions: How do I feel? What do I need? If you feel body hunger, you need to eat food! If you identify emotional hunger, you have needs that cannot be satisfied with food.

Take care of yourself. "Being healthy and fit is not just about how we treat ourselves the first two weeks of January," says registered dietitian Janice Harrell. "It's about being good to ourselves all through the year." Amen to that.

Focus on a healthful lifestyle, not just weight loss. "Work to be the very best person you can be," Harrell continues. "Put effort into treating others, and yourself, with fairness and kindness. Stand tall in the fact that your are loved for who you are and not how much you weigh. Embrace life and do the things that you really enjoy. Go for walks. Smell the flowers. Breathe the ocean breezes. Leave time for spontaneous fun."

Don't give up. As you set your expectations for this new year, consider this *Autobiography in Five Chapters* from the National Center of Mind and Science:

Chapter 1: I walk down the street. There is a deep hole in the sidewalk. I fall in. I am lost...I am helpless. It isn't my fault. It takes forever to find a way out.

Chapter 2 I walk down the same street. There is a deep hole in the sidewalk. I pretend I don't see it. I fall in again. I can't believe I am in the same place. But it isn't my fault. It takes a long time to climb out.

Chapter 3 I walk down the same street. There is a deep hole in the sidewalk. I see it is there. I fall in from habit. But my eyes are open. I know where I am. It is my fault. I get out immediately.

Barbara A. Quinn, MS, RD, CDE

Chapter 4 *I walk down the same street. There is a deep hole in the sidewalk. I walk around it.*

Chapter 5 *I walk down a different street.*

VALENTINE'S SURPRISES

It was Valentine's Day and I had a special date with my sweetie. When he showed up with a corsage of fresh flowers, I was convinced this was *the* evening. He drove us to a fine restaurant, where we were ushered to the best table. As he helped me settle into my chair, he asked, "Is this OK?"

Yes! I replied, practicing for the big question.

As we surveyed the menu in the romantic atmosphere, he leaned closer and asked, "Would you…like some wine?"

Yes! I blurted out anxiously.

As the evening wore on, I could feel our conversation becoming more romantic. Sure enough, at the end of our meal, his eyes met mine and he asked tenderly, "Would you…like some dessert?"

Yes, I sighed.

Still, it was a magical evening. We danced; we laughed; we talked. And then he drove me home and politely kissed me goodnight. And that…was it? Yes.

Valentine's Day is always full of surprises. And so is this day's special treat, chocolate. (Yes!) Made from cocoa beans that grow on *Theobroma cacao* trees, chocolate contains minerals like magnesium, copper, iron, and zinc. It also provides many of the same heart-protective antioxidant compounds found in tea and red wine. These "polyphenols" appear to help neutralize LDL cholesterol, the bad stuff that tends to clog arteries. A 1.5-ounce chocolate bar contains a similar amount of these polyphenols as a glass of red wine, say researchers. And dark chocolate contains twice as many polyphenols as milk chocolate.

But eating chocolate to lower your cholesterol would be like booking a ticket on the Titanic to learn how to swim. Don't forget that along with the beneficial substances in cocoa comes extra fat and calories. Yet not all the fat in chocolate is bad. About a third of the fat in cocoa butter is oleic acid, the same healthful monounsaturated fat found in olive oil. Another third is stearic acid, a saturated fat that does not raise blood cholesterol like other types of saturated fats. Stearic acid is not especially good for your heart; but it's not particularly harmful either.

And no, chocolate is not addictive, say researchers who know this because they study and eat chocolate every day, day in and day out. They say we eat chocolate because we desire the sensation of eating this delightfully sweet and creamy delicacy and not because it is physically addicting. And of course we can stop whenever we want to.

Chocolate may not be a major health food, say experts. But a little here and there can certainly be part of a healthy eating plan, according to nutrition experts. By the way, my sweetie did finally pop the question...two weeks later. And I said, "Yes."

GRANDMA QUINN'S IRISH SODA BREAD

Saint Patrick's Day is a big deal in our family. Invisible leprechauns sneak into the refrigerator and magically turn the milk green. We make corned beef and cabbage for dinner. And Grandma Quinn's Irish Soda bread tops off the meal.

This is not your typical soda bread. Grandma Quinn's is cake-like and a bit more sweet than salty. And her recipe, I was happy to discover, is healthful as well as delicious. At 80 calories per slice, it's low in fat (less than 2 grams), low in sodium (124 milligrams) and low in cholesterol (16 milligrams) even with real eggs in the recipe. And it's made with buttermilk which adds 60 milligrams of calcium per serving. This is the original recipe, as recorded by Annie Barry Quinn, Grandma Quinn's daughter:

Barbara A. Quinn, MS, RD, CDE

Grandma Quinn's Irish Soda Bread

Sift together: 2 cups flour, 1/2 cup sugar, 2 teaspoons baking powder, 1 teaspoon baking soda, and 1 teaspoon salt.

In separate bowl, beat together: 2 eggs, 2 cups buttermilk, and 2 tablespoons vegetable oil.

Mix the wet and dry ingredients together just until combined. (Raisins, currents and/or caraway seeds can be added at this step, if you prefer.)

Pour mixture into an oiled and floured loaf pan. Bake 55 to 60 minutes at 350 degrees F.

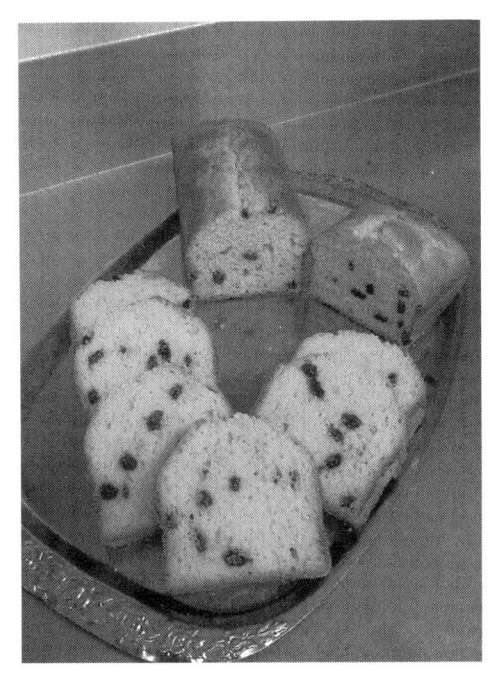

Grandmother Quinn's Irish Soda Bread

REFLECTION: Grandmother Quinn's grandson, Brian Quinn and his wife, Lisa, both graduates of the California Culinary Academy in San Francisco, prepare Saint Patricks' dinner for hundreds of people each year. Brian reports that Grandmother Quinn's Irish Soda Bread recipe is the highlight of their menu year after year.

"I have always thought that this can't be the actual recipe," Brian says. "It comes out more like a batter. Delicious? Absolutely! Crowd pleaser? Every time! As I remember it? Not really; the loaf I remember Grandma making was dry and rustic. Thank God for butter and jam for their rehydration properties! But it was made in love with Grandma's wrinkled and veined hands, served on a cake dish protected by a thin tea towel. It couldn't have been better!"

EGGS-CELLENT EASTER

Every year, even though our children are no longer children, I dye Easter eggs. And with a little prodding, a big Easter Bunny reluctantly hides eggs on Easter morning. Of course, we know that hens, not bunnies lay eggs. So here are some interesting facts from the *American Egg Board*:

- A hen can lay an egg every 24 to 36 hours. Thirty minutes after her egg is safe in the nest, Mrs. Hen begins the egg-making process all over again.
- Some hens produce eggs with two yolks. And on rare occasions, a hen may lay an egg with no yolk.
- Egg shells get their color from their parents. According to the *American Egg Board*, "The breed of hen determines the color of the shell. Among commercial breeds, hens with

- white feathers and ear lobes lay white-shelled eggs; hens with red feathers and ear lobes lay brown eggs."
- Egg yolks are colored by what a hen eats. Yellow-gold pigments in her feed such as marigold petals enhance the yellow color of the yolk. And by the way, no artificial color additives are permitted in chicken feed, notes the *American Egg Board*.
- Nutritionally, eggs are about as nutrient dense as you can get. Along with the 75 calories in one whole egg come these important nutrients:

Protein: With 4 grams in the white and 3 grams in the yolk, egg protein is the most complete and easily digestible mixture of protein building blocks (amino acids) on earth.

Vitamins A, D, and E: These nutrients are found in the yellow yolk. Eggs are one of the few natural food sources of vitamin D which is essential for a variety of body functions.

B-vitamins, including B-12 and folate: These critical nutrients preserve nerve and heart function.

Minerals: Eggs are natural sources of essential calcium, iron, and magnesium.

Omega-3 fatty acids: Especially in eggs from hens supplemented with flaxseed, canola, linseed and cod-liver oil, omega-3 fats have been shown to protect against heart disease and are essential for normal brain and visual development.

Cholesterol: One egg yolk typically contains 180 to 200 milligrams of dietary cholesterol, close to the 300 milligram daily limit set by the *American Heart Association* for healthy people. (For people with heart disease or diabetes, the goal for cholesterol is 200 milligrams per day.) However, research shows that cholesterol in the diet is not the major cause of elevated cholesterol in the blood stream. That honor is reserved for saturated fat, which is surprisingly low in eggs (about 1.5 grams per egg). If you have normal levels of blood cholesterol and no history of heart disease, most experts say you can enjoy eggs a few times a week. If you have diabetes or other risk factors for heart disease, however, you may need to limit egg yolks to no more than a couple a week.

Lastly, how in the world do all these nutrients find their way into a hard shell that grows into a baby chick as the moms sits on it? That is the miracle of Easter.

REFLECTION: One reader, poultry farmer Claude W. from Tampa, Florida, corrected an assumption that white eggs come from white-feathered hens and brown eggs from brown-feathered hens. He wrote, "I have raised poultry for some time. Some of my flock are White Cochin and they produce brown eggs." Indeed, it's not just the color of a hen's feathers but the color of her ear lobes that determines the color of her eggs, according to the McMurray Hatchery, experts in rare poultry breeds. Claude's White Cochin have white feathers and red earlobes; thus, they lay brown eggs. Mystery solved.

KENTUCKY DERBY PARTY

Odds are slim that you will ever feel hungry after a visit to Madge and Forrest's home. This is especially true if you participate in their annual Kentucky Derby party. These two are Kentucky-born and bred, after all. And you can bet they know how to feed a crowd.

Everything, and I mean everything, is Derby-themed in Madge's home on this day in May. Horsey pillows and pictures greet guests as we arrive in big hats and other Run-for-the-Roses

Barbara A. Quinn, MS, RD, CDE

Derby-wear. As we make our way to the back sunporch, Forrest offers guests mint juleps (with or without alcohol) garnished with freshly picked mint from their garden. As we sip our juleps, we are invited to pick a number for a winning horse from an authentic jockey's cap. This, my friends, is horse racing at its finest.

As we gather around a table saddled with Southern delicacies, Forrest says grace and thanks God for friends and family and food. I would run a mile and a quarter through the mud for this prized meal. Amid a spray of red roses, Madge's table groans with Kentucky fried chicken, country ham and biscuits, Kentucky Burgoo (a stew mixture of chicken, pork and beef), a colorful parade of fruit and vegetable salads and the best yeast rolls this side of Paintville, Kentucky.

"I'll give you the recipes," Madge offers in her it's-no-big-deal-to-prepare-a-feast-like-this-single-handedly style.

Later, down the straightaway comes Strawberry shortcake followed closely by Derby Pie, which I would describe as pecan and chocolate pie on steroids. Behind these are chocolate cake, and walnut pies; and assorted cookies are still in the race.

As I savor every crumb on my plate, I have an encouraging conversation with Madge and Forrest's daughter, Nina. This young lady suffers with a rare lung condition making breathing a struggle. She is unable to exercise and takes medications that thwart most efforts at weight control. Yet, on the advice of her doctor, this strong young woman has lost a significant amount of weight. How did she bridle her appetite under such competition?

"I've done the diet thing before," she tells me. "Where you eat only watermelon or some such thing and finally just get tired of it. It doesn't work."

What worked this time? I ask. "I realized, with all my limitations, food was my comfort. And so now I really like spinach. I really like it! And I like the little muffins that mom makes. I have one each morning for breakfast, just one. And once a week, I allow myself to have one slice, just one, of pizza. Knowing I can have some foods I really like makes me want to keep doing this."

And what about today? I ask. "My body hasn't had food like this in a long time," she says calmly. "And it really tastes good. But my stomach doesn't want me to eat as much as I once did. And I'm OK with that. I'll go home tonight and say, 'That was a nice meal.' And I'll just keep doing what I've done. Because I want to."

When the race is over and I accept the fact that my horse came in dead last, we were out the gate with well-fed tummies, minds, and spirits, and a souvenir glass commemorating this running of the Derby. Thank you, Forrest and Madge. You truly are a winning combination.

REFLECTION: In early 2015, Madge and Forrest's daughter, Nina, underwent successful lung transplant surgery. She continues to eat and exercise sensibly, even on Kentucky Derby day.

FACTS ABOUT THE GREAT PUMPKIN

How did I get to this point? I asked myself as I added eggs and nuts to a recipe for pumpkin bars. It started slowly, I suppose… my craving for pumpkin products. Yet more and more, I succumb to their temptings. It was innocent enough at first; a taste of pumpkin soup here, a pumpkin cookie there. But slowly, after each indulgence, I found myself attracted more and more. I sipped my pumpkin latte and thought about it.

This addiction is not entirely my fault; temptations are everywhere. Just last week as I stood in line to pay for pumpkin crackers, pumpkin butter and pumpkin body lotion, I admitted to the checker that I tend to overindulge on pumpkin items this time of year.

Barbara A. Quinn, MS, RD, CDE

"Oh you haven't even touched the surface," she assured me. "Did you see the pumpkin bagels and pumpkin cream cheese?" No, I didn't…

"And the pumpkin muffins are fabulous!" I had to confess these had been in my basket, but in a moment of repentance, I had put them back on the shelf. What is it that has me so enamored with pumpkins? A little research was in order.

Pumpkins have been around for centuries and appear to have originated in America, I learned. Native Americans ate pumpkins long before the colonists discovered them, say historians. A website on the topic from the University of Illinois Extension service says these large melons get their name from the Greek word "pepon" which means "large melon."

We tend to call them vegetables but pumpkins are really seed-bearing fruits, say experts. Pumpkins are related to cantaloupe, honeydew, and watermelon as well as squash and cucumbers. And they get their dense orange color from beta carotene, a powerful antioxidant that protects the eyes from macular degeneration, a serious eye disease. Beta carotene may also help protect against breast and ovarian cancers.

Nutritionally, my dear pumpkin is wonderfully dense in nutrients. According to the University of California at Davis Vegetable Research and Information Center, 1/2 cup of canned pumpkin contains about 40 calories and packs a good dose of protein, fiber, calcium, iron, zinc, and vitamins A, C, and E.

Pumpkin pie, say historians, originated with our colonist relatives (perhaps my great-great grandmother). Someone anyway, had the great idea to slice off the stemmed top, remove the seeds, and fill the pumpkin's cavity with milk, honey, and spices. This crustless "pie" was then baked over hot ashes.

While my pumpkin bars baked, I rearranged some pumpkins on the porch and realized that these bright cheery melons, and the food they provide, nourish my soul as well as my body. Maybe I'll sprinkle a little pumpkin pie spice on my coffee in the morning.

REFLECTION: Some say the idea of carved pumpkins started in Ireland. An Irish folktale tells of a fellow named Stingy Jack who was so despicable that God would not let him into heaven when he died. The devil didn't want him at his place either. So Jack was sent out into the night with only a burning coal to light his way. He put the coal into a carved out turnip and began to roam the earth which has nothing to do with nutrition but I might as well finish the story. The Irish refer to this homeless apparition as "Jack of the Lantern" which gave way to "Jack-o-lantern." Immigrants to the United States soon discovered that pumpkins made better jack-o-lanterns than turnips. And the rest is history.

TRICKS WITH HALLOWEEN TREATS

It's tricky, feeding kids. We want them to have fun and we want them to be healthy. Overindulge them on high-calorie sugar-laden treats and their health will suffer. Restrict them too much and as soon as they are off our radar screen, they go hog wild. So what do we do with Halloween? Take the middle ground, suggests registered dietitian and child feeding expert, Ellyn Satter. She offers this common sense advice:

- Use Halloween to help your child learn reasonable eating habits. "When he comes home from trick or treating, let him lay out his booty, gloat over it, sort it, and eat as much of it as he wants," Satter suggests in her book, *Your Child's Weight, Helping without Harming*. Let him do this for a day or two; then put the stash away and reserve it for appropriate times.
- Include Halloween candy in meals or snacks. To make this work, understand that snacks are more than treats

- or rewards. They are little meals for your child and thus should be presented reliably (at regular intervals) and matter-of-factly. And here's the clincher: Have your child sit at a table to eat snacks, not in her room or in front of the computer or television.
- Concentrate on structure. Sure, an apple with peanut butter is a much healthier snack than a Snickers bar. Yet children learn to regulate their intake of all foods when they are provided at specific meal and snack times.
- Treat Halloween treats as "controlled substances" instead of "forbidden fruit." Have a strategy to manage those wonderfully appealing, appallingly high calorie foods, says Satter. Overly restricting fun food can backfire and drive a child to overeat.

If your child can follow these rules, allow her to control her stash, says Satter. Otherwise, you control it. If you are doing a good job of providing regular meals and snacks to your child, a few days of eating candy will not impair her nutritional health, she assures us. And if you are *not* providing regular meals and snacks, all the candy restrictions in the world will not help much.

So how do we keep Junior from bouncing off the walls from eating too much sugar? "There is no reliable evidence that eating sugar causes children to have behavior problems," says Satter. However, eating sweets instead of something more substantial will leave a child nutritionally empty and cranky. That's one reason why we should offer goodies along with other, more nutritious foods during meal or snack times. These better foods can keep Junior comfortable until the next feeding time, she says.

HOW TO GAIN WEIGHT OVER THE HOLIDAYS

This is truly a special time, I thought as I sipped apple cider and munched on freshly baked goodies at a recent holiday event. Almost every occasion this month will be accompanied by delicious and

Quinn-Essential Nutrition

special foods that evoke fond memories of Christmases past; and that's good. But are these indulgences truly worth the extra pounds come January? If so, here is your plan:

- When you bake holiday cookies, eat one or two from each batch, just to make sure they are the way you remember them. And keep more at home than you give to friends and family, in case you get nostalgic in the middle of the night.
- At a holiday party, camp out at the buffet table. Fill your plate several times. And avoid anything that contains vegetables.
- When snacking on appetizers, load each cracker with a thick layer of cheese and dip.
- Refuse to eat anything but dark meat on the turkey and make sure you eat the skin, too. This choice contains three times more fat and a third more calories than light meat without the skin.
- Eat until you feel really full and uncomfortable. This will help you remember your holiday meal for days to come.
- On the morning of your big holiday function, have coffee for breakfast and skip lunch. Then you can ravenously anticipate everything you will devour at the party.
- To stay in the holiday spirit, have a large glass of eggnog, which weighs in at a cool 350 calories per cup, every night before going to bed. And grab a few cookies, too.
- Avoid any unnecessary physical activity over the holidays. Who has time anyway, when you're busy honking your horn at the car that took the space where you wanted to park close to the mall?
- Throw any thought of moderation out the window. When your coworker gives you a plate of homemade cookies, eat all of them on your drive home from work.
- Don't just sip on a nice glass of 75-calorie champagne. Splurge on a fancy cocktail that typically supplies at least 200 calories.

- When offered dessert, insist on the largest piece that will fit on your plate. And plop on an extra dollop of whipped cream, just because it's the holiday!

On the other hand, if you do *not* care to accumulate extra poundage over the holidays, ignore this list. Who knows? You may find that eating a little less makes you appreciate the season that much more.

THANKSGIVING A FUNCTIONAL HOLIDAY

Historians tell us that, before the first travelers to the New World boarded the Mayflower, they were instructed, "First, make thy will." Hopefully, we will not require the same from our Thanksgiving guests. Still, it's important to remember why we celebrate this holiday. That first Thanksgiving was not one of groaning from too much turkey and weird relatives. Rather, it was a thankful reprieve from the harsh reality of hunger and death that took the lives of more than half the Pilgrims during their first winter in this new country.

As we travel to be with loved ones this holiday, I am reminded that food has functions beyond nutrients. My daughter's homemade pies for example, mean more to us than the gazillion calories they contain. They crown our traditional holiday meal and offer an excellent excuse to head out for a walk while the guys clean up the kitchen.

Other foods we enjoy during this holiday are considered "functional" because they offer health benefits beyond their nutrient content. Cranberries are a good example. Besides looking nice with turkey, these tart little berries are storehouses of active substances that help the body fight the ravages of life, says registered dietitian Eileen Olmstead.

Some compounds in cranberries help prevent dental plaque from sticking to tooth surfaces. Others ward off the growth of *Heliobacter pylori,* unfriendly bacteria that can cause stomach ulcers. Cranberries also contain natural substances that protect against bladder infections; other compounds have been found to inhibit the growth of certain types of cancer. These benefits have been observed with an intake of about 10 ounces of cranberry juice a day, one-half cup of cranberry sauce or one ounce (about one-fourth cup) of dried cranberries.

So Thanksgiving may truly be a functional holiday. Special food shared with family and friends helps us endure the shocks of this world. And even though this is the season to count our blessings more than calories, we still need to be mindful not to overindulge on food *or* relatives.

Challenging life events could not shake the resolve of the early Pilgrims. They thanked God on that first Thanksgiving for the provision of life-sustaining food and friends in the midst of harsh realities. May we all do the same. Pass the dressing, please.

VINTNERS' HOLIDAY

One was described as "soft, round, and voluptuous." Another had "a lot of personality" and "great body." And to think my husband brought me to this place.

It was the Vintner's Holiday at the Ahwahnee Hotel in Yosemite, California. For two days, we learned the finer points of enology, the study of winemaking. We sniffed and sipped our way through reds, whites, and sparkling wines. One woman's tee shirt announced to the world, "Forgive me for I have Zinned."

Does wine have any redeeming value besides the fact that people love to study its complex tastes? It depends on what and how we drink, say health experts. For example, wine contains phenolic compounds that appear to block the destructive artery-clogging action of LDL "bad" cholesterol. When LDL becomes oxidized, it can build up in blood vessels, which is not good. Phenols in wine act as anti-oxidants that help to prevent the build-up of cholesterol in the arteries.

Most of these beneficial substances are found in the skins and seeds of grapes. And since red wine gets more skin contact in the winemaking process, it's the reds that have more phenols than the whites. In studies where volunteers drank red wine, researchers found fewer oxidized LDL particles in their blood. People who drank white wine had more of these not-so-good LDL's.

Heart disease is one thing. What about cancer? The *American Institute of Cancer Research* (AICR) says alcohol is a "human carcinogen" (capable of causing cancer). Excessive intake of alcohol, including wine, is related to cancers of the mouth, esophagus, and stomach. However, cancer experts go on to say, "current research suggests that people who eat healthy diets and do not smoke will probably *not* increase their cancer risk from moderate alcohol consumption."

Moderate is the key word here. Scientists have found that the curve from healthful imbibing to harmful drinking rises rapidly when women have more than one drink a day and men have more than two. And no, a mega 16-ounce glass of wine is *not* "one drink." Experts define one alcoholic beverage as 5 ounces of wine, 12 ounces of beer, or 1.25 ounces of spirits.

How moderate can you be at a vintner's holiday? Experienced wine masters at the daily seminars politely expelled most of the wine they tasted into an empty glass. The rest of us rookies were wise to heed the ancient advice, "Excellence resides in quality, not in quantity. Much lowers value."

COOKIE EXCHANGE

"So what do you do for a living?" the woman sitting next to me at the cookie exchanged asked. I'm a registered dietitian, I mumbled, wondering if she would believe me if I told her I was only there to conduct research.

Each year around this time, we women show up with two dozen of our favorite homemade cookies. After a festive dinner and a few rounds of Christmas carols, we exchange our cookies for a two-dozen assortment to take home.

Why do we have such a fascination for sweets? Blame it on our ancestors. A taste for sugar appears to be something we are born with, and probably for good reason. Milk, our first food, is naturally sweet with a simple sugar called lactose. Perhaps, say experts, babies are coaxed to their first nourishment by the sweet taste of mother's milk. I am well beyond my baby stage and I still crave the taste of sweets. Here are some more interesting facts about this food we call "sugar":

- Sugar is the basic building block of all carbohydrates, the body's primary fuel sources. Many types of sugar exist in nature. Glucose is the most common sugar in plants. Fructose is found primarily in fruit. One molecule of glucose combined with one molecule of fructose makes sucrose, or table sugar.
- Sugar does more than just taste sweet. It contributes to the soft brown texture of baked goods. And without it, your Christmas toffee will not caramelize.
- Measure for measure, sugar has fewer calories than fat. One teaspoon of sugar, for example, has 16 calories. A teaspoon of butter has 45 calories.
- Bacteria love sugar, too. That's why people with uncontrolled diabetes (high blood sugars) are prone to infections. Sugar also feeds bad bugs in our mouths that cause tooth decay.
- Sugar has some copy cats. My friend, Sheri has diabetes so she makes her Christmas cookies with a product called *Splenda,* which is also called *sucralose.* Six-hundred times sweeter than sugar, this sweetener retains its sweetness even at high cooking temperatures. Almost none is absorbed into the body so it does not raise blood sugar or insulin levels.
- Sugar alcohols with names like sorbitol, mannitol, and xylitol, are not really sugars and are not really alcohol.

They are carbohydrates that the body does not completely digest; thus they contribute fewer calories and carbs than other sugars. They can contribute to bloating, gas, and diarrhea, however, if we consume too many goodies made with them.

One last word of caution: Sugar tends to evaporate. I experience it every year when I get home with my two dozen delectable confections. The next morning, a few have inevitably disappeared.

REFLECTION: Our yearly cookie exchange is alive and well. And these new sweeteners have been approved by the Food and Drug Administration (FDA) for use by most people, including children, pregnant and breastfeeding women and people with diabetes:

- *Stevia (stevia rebaudiana) is a plant native to Central and South America. Extracts called steviol glycosides from the leaves of this plant are naturally sweet, and because we humans do not possess enzymes to digest these substances, they contribute sweetness with no calories. The words stevia extract, rebiana, or Reb A on a food ingredient label indicate the presence of stevia. Brand names include Truvia, Pure Via, and SweetLeaf.*
- *Monk Fruit is a green melon from South East Asia that got its name because it was used by monks. Compounds in this fruit called mogrosides are 150 to 200 times sweeter than sugar, so very small amounts are needed to sweeten food. Monk fruit sweeteners are considered calorie-free and have no effect on blood sugars. Look for words like monk fruit extract, luo han fruit, or luo han guo on products that use this sweetener; it also goes by the brand name, Nectresse.*

Quinn-Essential Nutrition

THE WEEK BEFORE CHRISTMAS POEM

My apologies to Clement Clarke Moore, who penned the famous poem, "The Night Before Christmas." This is my version:

The week before Christmas and all through our home,
Our family prepared for the big day to come.
Our cookies were baked with love and good cheer,
In hopes that they'd last 'til our company was here.
Icicles tacked on the roof line hung on,
As we prayed that the big storm soon would be gone.

And Dad in his pick-up and I in my van,
Had no time to eat right and nor did our clan.
We grabbed here and there and ate late in the night,
My plan for good eating was nowhere in sight.
A meal here and there plus a soda or two,
Made each of us know we had nutrients due.
Now soybeans, high fiber, omega and flax
Had gone from our diets like yesterday's trash.

Then out in the kitchen there arose such a clatter,
I stopped eating my cookie to see what was the matter.
When what to my malnourished eyes should appear
But bags full of food groups with value so dear.
A glass filled with milk and some bread of whole wheat,
Made me know in a moment this was my kind of treat.
A fresh cut-up orange and some nuts on the side,
It was now that I realized my health could not hide.
How enticing they took me away from the fudge,
And sparked up my fitness without extra pudge.
Now fresh fruit, now carrots, now veggies and greens,
Are full of nutrition but won't fill my jeans.

The message was clear as I put them away,
Keep your mind on good choices and balance each day.

Barbara A. Quinn, MS, RD, CDE

Less eggnog, more produce and sharing of food,
Small portions of goodies to make you feel good.
Choose whole grains and fresh food as part of my meal,
Choose cocktails with caution, gulp water with zeal.
Make merry with small sips of wine, not too much,
And walk some on most days for an energy rush.
As I got back to work, I had nothing to fear,
Not even the ads for chips, dips and beer,
And I realized the reason for Christmas is true,
Be wise and be loving whatever you do.
It's not about Santa or candy or gold,
But the message that wise men and angels behold.
I remembered these words as the days rolled away,
"It's a very good time for a fresh holiday!"

EATING STYLES

NUTRITION FOR ONE

My mother just loved having a dietitian for a daughter. Each time I came to New Mexico to visit, she got quizzed on her eating habits. Especially after my dad passed on and she ate most of her meals alone, I was even more persistent about her nutrition.

"It's not fun to eat alone, so I snack," she confessed.

No problem, I said. As long as your snacks provide the same nutrients you would have gotten in a balanced meal.

"What does that mean?" she asked.

It means, you can count a snack as a meal if it includes at least three of the five main nutrient categories: protein, milk (which includes cheese or yogurt); vegetables, fruit, and grains, preferably whole grains like cereal, bread, or crackers.

"Give me an example," she said.

A slice of your favorite melon with yogurt and a handful of whole wheat crackers qualifies as meal; three bags of popcorn do not.

"I can do that," Mom said.

What else is a challenge about eating alone? I asked.

"Sometimes I just forget to eat," she admitted. "I have a banana for breakfast and may not have anything else until late in the afternoon."

I frowned and asked her to suggest a solution for this nutritional no-no.

"Well," she thought, "if I'm out running errands, I can stop and have a balanced meal at a restaurant. Or I'll make myself a smoothie with fruit, milk, and an instant breakfast powder."

I concurred with her plan and asked her what type of supplements she was taking.

"Just a vitamin and mineral supplement for people over the age of 50," she said. I checked the label and saw that it included reasonable doses of essential vitamins and minerals; and it was formulated for older adults. I nodded my approval

Mom then looked at the clock and pretended to be serious. "Isn't there something else I should do to make sure I'm getting a balanced diet when you are here?"

Of course there is, I said with a smile. I grabbed the car keys and reminded her that, whenever I visited from California, we always had to go to Padilla's restaurant for green chile enchiladas. It's highly recommended by Native New Mexican dietitians.

LAND OF ENCHANTMENT

Oh fair New Mexico; we love we love you so.
Our hearts with pride o'erflow; no matter where we go...

I learned our state song when I was in the fourth grade at Collette Park Elementary School in Albuquerque, New Mexico. During a recent visit home, I found the words still ring true. What makes my native state so fair?

The weather. Whatever weather you like, you'll find it here. Bright blue skies, puffy white clouds, wind, thunderstorms, and sometimes it all comes in the same afternoon.

The food. Repeat after me, "sopapillas" (so-pa-PEA-yas). These little fried puffs of dough are standard additions to any real New Mexican restaurant. Eat 'em with the honey that sits on the table or else everyone will know you're a tourist.

The chile. Get used to it; when you order traditional New Mexican fare, your server will ask, "red or green?" Translation: Do you want your meal smothered with red chile or green chile? Both colors come from the same chile plant, according to my nephew Coye, a horticulturist in New Mexico. "Green chile is picked earlier in the season," he explains. "Red chile is the second harvest and has developed more sugar in the fruit. That's why red is usually not as hot as green.

And speaking of hot, chile gets its kick from a very active substance called "capsaicin" (cap-SAY-sin). This natural ingredient in chile can initiate healing reactions in the body, say experts. Here are some findings:

- In addition to sending messages to your brain that say, "Yikes! My mouth is on fire!" the sensory receptors activated by hot chile also release substances in the body that help relax pressure on blood vessels.
- Chile extract has been found to act like an antibiotic against *Heliobacter pylori,* the bacteria implicated as one cause of gastric ulcers;
- Contrary to what we might think, a randomized controlled research trial on 84 healthy people found that capsaicin *decreased* the amount of acid the stomach produced and *protected* the lining of the stomach;
- Hot chile may actually help you sweat off a few extra calories through a process called "thermogenesis." Some studies show that ingesting hot chile peppers revs up the body's calorie-burning machinery. Still no proof, however, that downing a plate of green chile enchiladas with a cold beer will help you lose weight.
- Topical skin creams that contain capsaicin help ease nerve pain caused by diabetes and other disorders, say scientists. Just don't rub it near your eyes!
- Researchers are still debating if chile helps reduce cancer risk. Some experts theorize that chile can irritate the stomach and lead to cancer. But the weight of evidence

suggests the opposite, according to one review on the subject. Capsaicin increases the rate of apoptosis, a process that makes cancer cells commit suicide. Caution is advised, however. Hot chile and spices can aggravate stomach conditions such as gastroesophagael reflux disease (GERD).

REFLECTION: The Chile Pepper Institute at New Mexico State University (my alma mater) reports than chile peppers are a nutrient dense food. One half cup of raw green chile (enough to really spice up your life) is loaded with vitamins A and C and contains healthy doses of folate, magnesium, zinc, and potassium. Phytonutrients are blazing in chile as well, including beta carotene, lutein and zeaxanthin. And yes, that hot thermal eruption we feel when we eat chile really does help burn off a few extra calories.

MEDITERRANEAN DIET

After watching the Summer Olympics in Athens, Greece, I reflected on what I learned from commentators and commercials over those weeks:

"His carbs are gone, and so is his Olympic dream." It wasn't low-carb beer that fueled these Olympic Games. It was glucose, the body fuel derived from carbohydrate-containing foods like pasta, rice, bread, fruit and juice. Nutrition researchers report that the higher an athlete's diet is in carbohydrates, the longer he or she can compete before becoming exhausted.

"I don't think this is going to be good enough." Carbs do not tell the whole story of athletic prowess, however. Exercise causes the body to tear down old cells and build new muscle structures, a process that requires adequate amounts of protein from foods such as fish, poultry, meat, milk, yogurt, beans and nuts.

"She's really struggling." Female competitors face unique challenges in their pursuit of sport greatness. The "female athlete triad" describes three dangerous health consequences when a woman jock eats poorly and exercises excessively:

1. Bizarre, disordered eating from her attempts to maintain an unrealistic weight for competition;
2. Loss of menstrual periods from eating a diet inadequate for her high level of exercise;
3. Weakened bones and stress fractures as a result of low estrogen levels and messed up menstrual cycles.

All these complications can be avoided or overcome when a female athlete eats a diet adequate for the activity she performs.

"She is a heavy favorite." Strongly muscled athletes may actually weigh more than their less fit peers. It's not the weight that matters; it's the composition of that weight.

"The nice thing about this routine is there is a lot of variety." Indeed, if eating were an Olympic event, the Mediterranean people would win the gold for style and form. Although this pattern of eating varies from region to region, people of Greece and other Mediterranean countries seem to have found one of the healthiest routines in the world. Here are the key components of this diet:

- Olive oil is rich in oleic acid, a monounsaturated fat that can help prevent a type of internal inflammation associated with heart disease. Studies have found that when olive oil is eaten in place of more saturated types of fats, it can

reduce the level of LDL "lousy" cholesterol and maintain "healthy" HDL cholesterol in the blood.
- Grains, especially whole grains in pasta, polenta, couscous and rice. These carbohydrates fire up the brain and fuel active muscles.
- Fruits and vegetables. Mediterranean people enjoy simply prepared, fresh, seasonal produce with meals. Fruit is eaten often for dessert.
- Beans, lentils and nuts provide cholesterol-lowering fiber that is often missing in American fast food fare.
- Fish, eggs, poultry, meat in small portions is the general order of preference for protein foods in Mediterranean countries.
- Dairy foods such as cheese and yogurt, are included with meals to provide essential protein and calcium.
- Wine is consumed with meals in moderation.

Exercise is a daily routine for our Mediterranean neighbors. Meals are not slammed down while driving in rush hour. Rather it is savored, shared and enjoyed with others. That's a truly winning routine, say experts.

REFLECTION: Evidence continues to accumulate on the health effects of the Mediterranean style of eating. In 2013, an observational study on 10,670 women in their 50's and 60's found that those who ate more plant-based foods, whole grains, and fish, less red and processed meats, and limited alcohol were 40% more likely to live past the age of 70 with no chronic illness and fewer physical and mental problems than those with less healthful diets.

Other reviews show that the Mediterranean diet may slow mental decline as we age. In some studies, subjects who adhered to this dietary pattern were better able to remember details and manage their time when compared to those on a typical western diet.

EATING VEGETARIAN

So, your son tells you he won't eat anything with a face. Or your daughter refuses to ingest food that once had a mother. Should you worry? Depends. According to a position paper on vegetarian diets from the *Academy of Nutrition and Dietetics*, vegetarian diets are appropriate and healthful choices for adolescents, if they receive guidance in planning meals. Here's how to do that:

Know what is missing. Some vegetarian eating styles are easy to manage nutritionally. Others eliminate major nutrient groups and can be more challenging.

"Semi-vegetarians," for example, may eat little or no red meat, a significant source of blood-building iron and growth enhancing zinc. This group may eat poultry, eggs or fish on occasion. And they usually consume dairy foods which provide a bulk of protein, calcium and vitamin D to the diet. Jump for joy if your teen wants to follow this type of vegetarian diet. It can be easily planned to include all essential nutrients for growth and development.

"Pesco-vegetarians" eat no animal food except fish, eggs, and milk products. Depending on how well it is planned, this type of diet may require alternate sources of iron and zinc.

"Lacto-ovo-vegetarians" exclude all animal foods except milk products "lacto" and eggs "ovo." Adolescent athletes who eat this way need special attention to get enough iron, zinc, protein and calories. Research shows that lacto-ovo vegetarians may also become deficient in vitamin B-12 which keeps nerve and blood cells healthy and is used to make the genetic material, DNA.

"Vegan" diets exclude any food even remotely associated with animals. Only foods from plant sources such as fruit, vegetables, grains, seeds, beans, and nuts are consumed. By far, this is the most challenging vegetarian diet for growing teens. Nutrients at risk of being deficient include calcium, iron, protein, zinc, and calories.

Find plant-based substitutes. Here are some examples:

Protein: Most vegetarian diets supply enough protein if they supply adequate calories. (When enough calories are consumed, protein is spared for its more important body functions.) Protein is found in milk, eggs, nuts, beans, grains, and yes, even vegetables. And we can disregard the old notion that two incomplete plant proteins--such as beans and rice—are only beneficial if eaten at the same meal. Just make sure your teen gets a good variety of protein-containing foods throughout the day.

Calcium: Compare the calcium content of alternate foods to a cup of milk or yogurt which contain about 300 milligrams (mg) of calcium: 1 cup calcium-fortified orange juice, tofu, or soy milk (200 to 400 mg), 5 figs (250 mg), 1 tablespoon blackstrap molasses (185 mg), ½ cup cooked turnip or collard greens (150 mg), 1 cup cooked beans (125 mg). If these foods are not on your teen's nutritional radar, consider a supplement.

Iron: Popeye got his iron from spinach. It is also in seaweed, dried beans and peas, nuts and seeds, molasses, dried fruit and fortified breads and cereals. And he'd be smart to pop a can of orange juice along with the spinach since vitamin C helps the body absorb the type of iron found in plant foods. Examples of iron-containing teen foods: Bean (iron) burrito with tomatoes and salsa (vitamin C), cereal with raisins or molasses (iron), garbanzo beans and pumpkin seeds (iron) added to a tomato salad (vitamin C).

REFLECTION: Results in 2013 from an on-going study involving 96,469 Seventh-day Adventist men and women continues to support the health-enhancing effects of plant-based diets. Researchers for this Adventist Health Study-2 found a lower risk for death from all causes in vegetarians versus non-vegetarians. Interestingly, risk was generally lower for pescatarians (fish-eating vegetarians) than for strict vegetarians. Also of interest from this study: The incidence of metabolic syndrome, associated with heart disease and type 2 diabetes, was lower in vegetarians than non-vegetarians.

FAMILIES THAT EAT TOGETHER

I got a gentle reminder last week that I missed "A Day to Eat Dinner with Your Family." Not to worry, I was assured by Nancy Gavilanes of Columbia University, sponsor of this event. "We encourage families to eat together every day." They have good reasons to encourage us, according to a survey conducted by the National Center on Addiction and Substance Abuse (CASA) at Columbia University. Compared to teens who eat two or fewer dinners a week with their families, teens who eat dinner with their families at least five times a week are less likely to smoke cigarettes or try marijuana, less likely to try alcohol, more likely to get better grades in school and more likely to have parents who take responsibility for teen drug use.

What's the secret in simply eating a meal together? "Family dinners and the communication that occurs over the course of a meal are critical in building a relationship with your children.. and to understanding the world in which they live," says Joseph A. Califano, Jr. former U.S. Secretary of Health, Education and Welfare and chairman of CASA. "Parents who have frequent family dinners are those who take the time to know their child's friends and the parents of those friends. They know their chid's teachers and chaperone their parties. And they have healthier kids."

That's nice, but why don't we eat together more often? Too many conflicting schedules and parents that get home late, say parents and 12 to 17 year-olds who answered this survey. Here are some strategies to help us get back on track:

1. Make family meals a priority. Eat *with* our children, don't just feed them, says registered dietitian and child-feeding expert Ellyn Satter. Strive for regular meals on schedule most of the time.
2. Define your terms. A *family meal* is sitting at a table with other family members eating the same food. It does not include television, computers, or video games.

3. Keep it simple. Dump leftover chicken, ham, boiled eggs, beans, nuts, cheese, and whatever else you find in the fridge over a pile of lettuce and other vegetables. Serve with whole grain crackers and a glass of milk and voila! You have a fast and easy chef's salad dinner.
4. Know your own responsibilities. Parents are responsible for what food is prepared as well as when and where it is eaten. Children are responsible to sit at the table with the family to eat..or not.

"It's your table," stresses pediatric dietitian Kristina Eisaesser. Children learn eating patterns and food choices from you. It's OK *not* to cater to kids.

Lastly, have some ground rules. Even if you pick up a pizza on the way home, add a vegetable or salad and sit down together. It is well worth it.

LIVE TO EAT OR EAT TO LIVE?

My friend Cindy told me that one Thanksgiving, her family forgot to eat their holiday meal. "We just got busy doing other things," she said. "Towards the end of the day, we suddenly realized we hadn't made the meal yet."

That would *never* happen in the Quinn family. Our meal *is* our holiday. We order a special turkey. We plan the menu weeks ahead. I take out a loan to buy groceries. We are, what registered dietitian and child obesity expert Laurel Mellin, calls a "live to eat" family.

Cindy's family is the other extreme. Her family "eats to live," according to Mellin, who developed a child and adolescent weight management program called *Shapedown*. Food is not the center of the universe to these folks. It is simply something to consume when you get hungry.

Which is best? Neither, says Mellin. Somewhere in between is the best way to enjoy good food and maintain optimal health.

Quinn-Essential Nutrition

These questions will help you determine if you "live to eat" or "eat to live."

Do you:
>   A. Fantasize about cooking like a famous chef? or
>   B. Love recipes you can mix up in one bowl?
>   A. Remember everything you ate last Thanksgiving? or
>   B. Remember everything you did last Thanksgiving?
>   A. Relax when you cook? or
>   B. Relax when someone else cooks?

Could you:
>   A. Create a gourmet meal from leftovers? or
>   B. Enjoy a peanut butter sandwich for dinner?
>   A. Give up a hike in the mountains to make a special meal? or
>   B. Give up a special meal to take a hike in the mountains?

Holiday advice for "A's" who live to eat: Get your nose out of the turkey. Learn to shift some of your focus away from food and develop relationships with people instead. Enjoy a brisk walk instead of a second piece of pie.

For B's, who eat to live: Go ahead, open a cooking magazine. Try a new recipe. Use two bowls. Learn to enjoy the pleasure of a special meal.

And for all of us as we approach this day of thanks: Share your meal, however simple or sensational, with others. Savor the food you eat; enjoy each bite. Talk freely and listen attentively to one another as you eat. Do not discuss how many calories are in the dessert. And do not remind others of how much they should eat or not eat. Whether we eat to live or live to eat, we can be thankful for this food on this day.

REFLECTION: A reader named Bob thought this column was a bit too light-hearted. Here's what he wrote, which was featured in a subsequent piece:

"An important area that your article didn't get into is the friction that comes up when a person who eats to live spends time with a person who lives to eat."

"A prime example," he says, "is when a person who eats to live and a person who lives to eat are vacationing together. The person who eats to live will think the other person's meal plans are taking too much time away from other activities like hiking, fishing, kayaking, and sight-seeing. The person who lives to eat will think the other person's activity plans are taking too much time away from his or her meal plans."

"The person who eats to live will likely just pack some food items in a cooler and make a sandwich at a pull-out when he/she gets hungry," Bob continues. "The person who lives to eat will often want to drive a long ways out of the way to eat at a restaurant or go back to camp early to start cooking."

"The live-to-eat people won't want to start any of the day's activities until after they've have a big breakfast. And the eat-to-live people are more likely to do some recreation before their first meal of the day."

"Also," he says, "a person who eats to live will get bored around people who live to eat. If a BBQ is planned for the afternoon, an eat to live person will likely try to get some recreation like water skiing in that morning, so that they don't spend the entire day just eating and talking."

"All of these scenarios," Bob concludes, "can potentially lead to friction...and hopefully compromise."

Yes, they certainly can.

NAVAJO WAYS

I was cleaning out some old files and happened upon a folder labeled "Navajo Ways." In it were papers I had saved from my

Quinn-Essential Nutrition

first professional job, as the nutritionist for the Navajo Nation *HeadStart* preschool program.

How hard can it be? I remember thinking. I'd only be living and working for the largest Native American tribe in the United States, with boundaries that extend 27,000 square miles into New Mexico, Arizona and Utah. I was a young and energetic native New Mexican, used to wide open spaces. So I packed up and moved to Fort Defiance, Arizona, just outside the Navajo capital of Window Rock. I soon realized, however, that my real life education had just begun. These are the lessons I learned from my Navajo friends:

Seek to understand. My youthful vision of teaching families to stock their refrigerators with fresh food was dashed when I realized that few households on the reservation had electricity. I soon understood why most food was boiled or fried or cooked directly over hots coals.

Don't panic. Navajo words for hello "YAY-ta-eh" and thank you "Eh-HYEH-heh" were common. But there was no word in this native language for "nutrition." Food "chi-YAWN" was what you ate when you were hungry. Food to keep you healthy…that was a new concept.

Be creative. I drove a pick-up truck to and from my duties, as did most Navajo families. It was well understood that our vehicles needed gas, oil and water to run efficiently. And that became my analogy for nutrition—foods that provide high quality fuel and fluids for our bodies.

Be flexible. I was not particularly fond of mutton stew, which was heavy on old sheep and light on vegetables. Yet it was often the only dish offered at staff meetings and parent events. On these occasions, I learned to relax my nutrition standards in order to accept the hospitality of my hosts.

Try new foods. I did fall in love with Navajo tacos, which featured pinto beans, green chile, cheese, lettuce and tomatoes on a bed of traditional fried bread (I know, I know). I also justified that several nutrient groups were represented in this classic dish.

It's OK to say No. One day, my co-worker offered me a sample of her lunch—a roasted and green chile-stuffed prairie dog. I respectfully declined; and she understood.

Keep learning. In my Navajo files, I found an article from a 1976 issue of *Organic Gardening and Farming*. It describes how native Americans commonly cooked corn in water that had been sprinkled with ashes from their open fires. Later analyses showed that this practice increased the ability of nutrients like calcium, iron and magnesium to be absorbed by the body. Today, Navajo children, like other American youngsters, fall short on their intakes of calcium and iron-rich foods. And they over-consume sugar-sweetened drinks and high fat snacks. We still have much to learn.

READERS QUESTIONS

PALEO DIET

Q: "My daughter and her fiancé are on the Paleo diet most of the time. When they were here for a visit last week, they told my wife and I about it and it sounds pretty reasonable. What do you think?"

Dear Jim,

I recently reviewed this diet for another publication. Its basic premise is that we would all be healthier if we ate the same foods as our ancestors did 2.5 million years ago during the Paleolithic Era. Thus, this diet focuses on foods that can be hunted, fished or gathered such as wild game, meat, fish, nuts, berries, seeds, fruit and vegetables. Grains and legumes are prohibited because they were not introduced until the Neolithic period when food began to be cultivated and farmed. Dairy foods are out as well, since it was probably very difficult to milk prehistoric cows.

Supporters of the Paleo diet present evidence that our current diet destroys our caveman/cavewoman constitution. They point out studies that show how highly processed foods with added salt, sugar and fat have contributed to modern diseases like obesity, diabetes and heart disease. I cannot argue with that. I am not convinced, however, that trading my morning granola and yogurt for a grass-fed bison burger (hold the bun) is always the best choice. As you point out, many people who follow this diet can stay with it only "most of the time." I think it's always good to get back to basics. I'm just not sure I need to go back 2.5 million years.

Q: "Dear Barbara, I realize you aren't Ann Landers. However, I do have a family problem that is in your area of expertise. We've tried for several years to convince my granddaughter that several members of her family should diet and exercise. I've been rebuffed on each occasion and my suggestions are totally ignored. Now, my great granddaughter has changed from a beautiful child into a blimp. My family members live in another state which makes it more difficult for me. Do you have any written material that spells out the ghastly effects of childhood obesity? I'm out of ideas. Thanks for listening to my problems. Sincerely, Concerned Granddad"

Dear Concerned,

True, I'm not Ann Landers, but I can point you to materials that spell out the sad effects of childhood obesity. One is a report on childhood obesity from the US Centers for Disease Control and Prevention http://www.cdc.gov/obesity/childhood/problem.html

I also propose that your well-intentioned suggestions may not be the best solution for your family's weight issues. When defenses go up, motivation to make changes often goes down. I would guess that your great-granddaughter is a beautiful child and needs to hear that.

OF EGGS AND GRAINS

Q: "Regarding eggs, is the protein in the white different from that in the yolk?"

A: It is the same protein, generally referred to as albumin. The white of one large egg contains about 3.5 grams of protein; the yolk contains about 2.5 grams. One whole egg contains about the same amount of protein as one ounce meat, fish, or poultry. Egg protein is also a complete protein; it contains all the amino acids needed to manufacture any other protein required by the human body; and it's one of the most easily digested food proteins.

Q: "What other nutrients are found in eggs?"

A: Besides their reputation for being loaded with cholesterol—one egg yolk contains close to the daily limit for most of us— eggs are also rich in other nutrients.

Egg yolks contain linolenic acid, an omega-3 fatty acid essential for brain development in growing babies, both in and out of the womb. Other nutrients in egg yolks include vitamin B-12, calcium, iron and zinc. Egg yolks get their yellow color from lutein, a potent antioxidant that protects the eyes from sun damage and may help prevent a serious eye disease called macular degeneration.

Q: "What is the substance in eggs that causes allergic reactions in some people?"

A: Egg protein is responsible for allergic reactions in susceptible people. By the way, egg allergy is fairly common in young children with immature digestive systems.

Q: "How long can you safely store eggs?"

A: Three to five weeks if you refrigerate them properly, says a national food safety website, FoodSafety.gov. An egg's shell and the membrane just under the shell form natural barriers to protect unbroken eggs from harmful bacteria.

Q: "I eat whole grain breads 95 percent of the time, but I'm confused about what constitutes a 'whole grain.' Does cracked wheat count?"

Sure does. So do amaranth, buckwheat (also known as kasha), bulgur, millet, oat meal, quinoa, wheat berries, brown rice and wild rice. "Whole grain" means the entire part of the grain kernel is present in a food; this includes the bran (a source of fiber), the germ (a storehouse of vital nutrients), and the endosperm (the energy source). According to the United States Food and Drug Administration, a product can be labeled "whole grain" if at least

Barbara A. Quinn, MS, RD, CDE

51% of its ingredients are whole grain wheat, whole grain rye, whole grain corn...you get the picture.

Another interesting finding about grains: Nutrition scientists are studying sorghum, a nut-flavored grain used widely in animal feed, as an alternate grain for humans with celiac disease. Why? Sorghum is free of gluten, the protein that people with celiac disease must avoid.

MARGARINE

A man I once knew asserted that "interesting" was a a female word, one that women use when we don't necessarily agree with something.

"Guys never use that word," he said. "We'll say, 'That's the stupidest thing I've ever heard.' A woman will say, 'That's interesting."

That's interesting; and it reminds me of some curious statements I've heard recently about margarine. I've listed them here, along with the facts:

"Margarine was originally manufactured to fatten turkeys."

Margarine was formulated in 1869 by a French pharmacist in response to a contest held by Emperor Napoleon III to find a suitable replacement for butter.

"Butter has been around for centuries while margarine has been around for less than 100 years."

In 2013, the patent for margarine in the United States was 140 years old. It was used in Europe before it came to the US.

"Margarine and butter have the same amount of calories."

This is true, unless you use a lower fat version of either.

"Butter is slightly higher in saturated fat than margarine, 8 grams versus 5 grams per tablespoon."

Butter typically contains 7 or more grams of saturated fat per tablespoon. Most soft (tub or liquid) margarines contain about 2 grams or less of saturated fat.

"Eating margarine can increase heart disease in women by 53 percent over eating the same amount of butter, according to a recent Harvard Medical Study."

What this research really said was that women who ate four daily teaspoons of hard stick margarine (the kind that contains dangerous *trans* fats) had a 50 percent greater risk for heart disease than those who ate this type of margarine rarely. Very few margarines contain *trans* fats today, especially the softer tub margarines.

"Butter has many nutritional benefits where margarine has only a few."

Butter is 100 percent fat; so is margarine. They differ in the type of fat they contain. Butter is mostly saturated fat and contains cholesterol. Margarine is mostly unsaturated fat and contains no cholesterol. Stick-type margarines may also contain *trans* fats which have been implicated in heart disease and are being phased out of our food supply.

"Margarine is very high in *trans* fatty acids, substances that increase bad LDL cholesterol and lower good HDL cholesterol levels."

Read the label. Most soft (liquid or tub) margarines contain no *trans* fat.

"Margarine is one molecule away from being plastic."

And interestingly, water is one molecule away from being a strong acid. But I digress. Margarine is made from the same basic molecules as butter—carbon, hydrogen and oxygen. What differentiates one from the other is how these molecules are put together to form various types of fat.

"Avoid margarine for life and anything else that is hydrogenated."

In November 2013, the FDA began to phase *trans* fats (made from partially hydrogenated oils) out of our food supply based on evidence that higher intakes of these fats increased our risks for heart disease. Most soft margarine products are now free of *trans* fat. Small amounts might still be found in more solid margarines as well as packaged snack foods, frozen pies and pizzas.

KIDS WHO DON'T EAT MEAT

A reader writes: "We recently had a visit from our niece, her husband, and 12 year-old boy. We were surprised to find out that the father and son both eat no meat. We believe the boy should be eating from all the basic food groups and meat is one of them. Are we right, or should we just let nature take its course? The boy's mother is a life-long diabetic. Does this matter?

Dear Reader,

You are absolutely right that the boy should be eating from all the basic food groups. Meat, however, is not one of them. We are advised by health experts to build a diet from five nutrient groups: Protein, Grains, Fruits, Vegetables, and Dairy. Meat is in the "Protein" group, and so are fish, poultry, eggs, dry beans, nuts and seeds. All these foods can be interchanged to provide necessary protein.

A 12 year-old boy may choose to eat a soy burger instead of cheeseburger burger, for example. Or peanut butter on his sandwich instead of ham. He can also get high quality protein from milk, cheese, yogurt and eggs as well as poultry and fish. Most of us need to eat at least two servings of protein-rich foods each day.

It's true that meat is an excellent source of B-vitamins, including vitamin B-12 which is generally only found in animal-based foods. Meat such as beef and pork are also rich sources of zinc, iron and selenium. People who choose not to eat these foods can get these nutrients from other foods or supplements.

As for your last question, should you just let nature takes its course? You might find the following helpful:

3000 POUNDS OF PEANUT BUTTER LATER

I was delighted to hear back from a young man I had mentioned in a recent column. Several years ago when he was in elementary school, I met with him and his mother regarding his extremely limited diet; he would only eat peanut butter sandwiches, spinach and a few other foods.

Surprisingly, an analysis of his actual nutrient intake revealed that his basic needs were being met...at least for the short term. Not to worry about these temporary food jags, I advised his parents. Children usually outgrow these types of limited food preferences as they mature.

Fast forward twenty years when this letter arrived in my mail:

"Hello, Barbara! My mother sent me a copy of your article after she recognized that you were probably talking about me! I'm the one who only eats peanut butter, bread, spinach and apple sauce. I'll be 30 years old in December and I still eat pretty much the same way I did when we first met.

"I eat a peanut butter sandwich every day for lunch and dinner and I still eat spinach and apple sauce every night. Apparently the long term effects of eating this way aren't so bad either. I'm currently 6'1" and weigh 203 pounds, according to my bathroom scale, and I have no major health problems. I certainly could lose weight, but I'm working on it and making progress.

"My wonderful fiancee figured out how to get the peanut butter I eat in bulk and how much I actually eat. We kept track of my consumption over a few months and it turns out I eat a 26-ounce jar of Laura Scudder's All Natural Smooth Peanut Butter every five days on average. I've been eating this way for about 25 years, so if you use that average, I've eaten around 3,000 pounds of peanut butter over my lifetime.

"I'm amused you still remember me. I'm glad I saw your column so I could write and say, Hi. It is almost dinner time, so I had better go make myself a sandwich." F.Z.

CHIA AND ORANGE JUICE

Q: "I heard that chia seeds are higher in omega-3 fatty acids than flaxseeds. Is this correct?

A: Chia and flax seed have similar amounts of omega-3 fatty acids, according to data from the USDA National Agricultural Research Service (ARS). One ounce (about two tablespoons) of chia seeds contains 5 grams of alpha-linolenic acid (ALA), the plant form of omega-3 fat. One ounce of flaxseed contains 6.3 grams of ALA.

In the old days, chia was a cute little plant that you could grow to look like a pet and give to someone for Christmas. Today chia (botanical name *Salvia hispanica L.*) meets criteria as a "functional food," one that provides additional health benefits beyond its basic nutrient content.

Case in point: A small study of men and women with type 2 diabetes found that adding about three tablespoons of chia seeds to their usual diet for three months helped control their blood sugars and blood pressures. Another small study found that a diet rich in high fiber foods including chia seeds helped reduce the risk for developing heart disease and diabetes.

Beware of claims, however, that chia seeds contain "eight times more omega-3's than salmon". This is like saying that a team of horses contains more "horse" power than a diesel engine. Two types of omega-3 fatty acids exist in food, and their actions differ. Alpha-linolenic acid (ALA) is found in plants (including flax, walnuts, and chia). EPA (eicosapentaenoic acid) and DHA (docosahexaenoic acid) are the more active (and probably most beneficial) omega 3 fatty acids found in salmon and other fatty fish. Best bet: Eat foods that provide both types of healthful omega-3 fatty acids.

Quinn-Essential Nutrition

A reader in Oregon writes: "I have a question about the vitamin C content of prepared juice compared to frozen orange juice. I keep the juice in my refrigerator, and before I drink it, I warm it in my microwave. Do you think I am reducing the Vitamin C content by warming it?"

Dear Reader,
Vitamin C is indeed a sensitive nutrient; it tends to disappear when it comes in contact with air or heat. Experts recommend we store reconstituted orange juice in the refrigerator in a tightly covered container. If used within six days, reconstituted orange juice retains up to 80% of its vitamin C content. A bit of warming should not destroy vitamin C, as long as you don't heat your orange juice above 70 degrees F., say experts.

MUCUS AND INFLAMMATION

Best quote overheard this week: "I'm done with diets. I'm just going to eat sensibly."

Most interesting entry in a patient's diet history: "I cannot eat flower tortillas."

And here are some good questions from readers:

Q: "My 92 year-old husband is in generally good health. But he has an excessive amount of clear chest mucous which he expectorates fairly frequently. Could drinking four milkshakes a week, diluted with 2% milk, possibly be an influence? Your well written, sensible column is a reliable delight. Thank you." g.w.

A: Dear g.w.
A widely viewed belief is that milk makes mucus, although scientific studies have not shown this to be true. One study exposed volunteers to a cold virus, known to produce mucus. These volunteers were then instructed to drink up to 11 glasses of milk a day to see if the mucus production worsened. Scientists measured

the congestion and nasal secretions from each volunteer, which does not sound like fun. Results? Drinking milk did not increase or worsen the production of mucus in these subjects.

Although rare in adults, a runny nose could be a symptom of a milk allergy. Best way to find out? Lay off the milkshakes for a week or so and see if the symptoms resolve.

Q: "Is there a good diet to reduce inflammation in the body?"

A: Why yes, there is. But first, let's talk about inflammation. One type of inflammation produces pain, swelling, and heat as a result of infections or injuries. "Silent inflammation" is associated with chronic diseases such as heart disease, diabetes, arthritis, and Alzheimer's disease. Some foods and food components work against inflammation and are thus anti-inflammatory. Here are the basics:

- Eat a variety of colorful fruits and vegetables.
- Choose whole grains over refined grains.
- Consume omega-3 fatty acids from fish, flax, walnuts or fish oil supplements. Omega-3's have been shown to disrupt the signals that lead to inflammation.
- Avoid *trans* fats and eat less saturated fat; both are considered inflammatory fats. In their place, choose vegetable oils, nuts, seeds, and avocados. Olive oil, for example, contains a chemical called "oleocanthal" that acts similar to the non-steroidal anti-inflammatory medicine, ibuprofen.
- Eat less sugar. Drink less alcohol.
- Add spices to your life! Ginger and turmeric, found in curry powder, have anti-inflammatory qualities that guard against premature aging.

This anti-inflammatory way of eating is very similar to two other eating patterns, the Mediterranean diet and DASH (Dietary Approaches to Stop Hypertension), which are protective against heart disease and other chronic diseases. Remember too, that obesity is now considered an inflammatory condition (no pun intended).

REFLECTION: Chronic inflammation can also result from smoking, inadequate sleep, obesity, lack of exercise and eating too much saturated fat and sugar, say experts. This internal inflammatory response decreases the brain's ability to regenerate itself, speeding up the aging process.

A study in the 2014 Journal of the Academy of Nutrition and Dietetics reported that women who ate more cruciferous vegetables such as cabbage, broccoli, bok choy, brussels sprouts, kale and cauliflower had lower levels of inflammatory markers in their circulation. Cruciferous "cross-bearing" vegetables are named for their four-petal flowers that resemble a cross; and they contain antioxidant nutrients that fight oxidative stress, the cause of inflammation. These particular vegetables are also good sources of phytochemicals called isothiocyanates and indoles which have been found to inhibit tumor (cancer) growth in addition to their ant-inflammatory effects.

Cruciferous vegetables contain enzymes that may interfere with the formation of thyroid hormone but only at very high intakes. Cooking these vegetables significantly reduces these enzymes. Health experts recommend we eat two to three cups of cruciferous vegetables each week.

Omega-3 fats appear to have potent anti-inflammatory effects. Yet a 2013 study in the Journal of the National Cancer Institute found that men with high blood concentrations of long-chain omega-3 fatty acids (the kind found in fish oils) were at increased risk for prostate cancer. Scientists speculate that omega-3's may have properties not well understood and could perhaps cause oxidative stress at high doses. Until we understand more, it may be wise to follow the advice of the American Heart Association: Take no more than 3 grams (3000 milligrams) of omega-3 fatty acids unless you are under the care of a physician.

LACTOSE INTOLERANCE

Dear Barbara:

I wonder if you have any information about lactose intolerance. I realized last year (at the age of 52) that cutting back on dairy settled a lifelong jumpy stomach. Can you direct me to published resources for advice on this? —Jeanne

Dear Jeanne:

Lactose intolerance can surely make your stomach jumpy. Symptoms include cramps, gas and diarrhea. Lactose is the natural sugar in milk that normally is digested by an enzyme called "lactase." Many people do not produce sufficient amounts of lactase to fully digest lactose. An estimated 30 to 50 million Americans, especially those of African, Jewish, Native American, Hispanic and Asian descent, are lactose intolerant. Here are some strategies to help relieve your distress:

- Replace regular milk with lactose-free alternatives such as soy or almond milk; and make sure the substitute is enriched with calcium and vitamin D.
- Try small amounts of lactose-containing foods with other foods. Many people can tolerate milk products this way. As you gradually increase your intake of lactose, your body can begin to manufacture additional lactase enzymes.
- Try low lactose dairy foods, such as *Lactaid*, a milk product to which the lactase enzyme has been added. Yogurt contains about half the lactose of milk. And cheese contains very low amounts of lactose compared to milk.

- Do not confuse lactose intolerance with a true milk allergy, which involves an allergic reaction to milk proteins. In the case of allergies, *all* dairy foods are no-no's.
- Lastly, find reliable published resources from the National Institutes of Health, National Digestive Diseases Information Clearinghouse (NIH-NDDIC): http://digestive.niddk.nih.gov/ddiseases/pubs/lactoseintolerance/

UNFERMENTED SOY

"Could you help me figure this out?" a reader asks. "An article in a local newsletter said to avoid 'non-fermented soy' which can place a multitude of health risks on yourself and your family. I buy organic soy milk and the carton does not mention fermentation on the carton. Would you please let me know what I should do?"

Don't panic. There's a lot to be paranoid about these days, but non-fermented soy milk is not on the list. Here are some facts:

Soybeans are high-protein legumes, highest in protein quality of any plant protein, in fact. A variety of foods come from soybeans, such as tofu (soybean curd), soy milk (liquid extracted from soybeans), and fermented products like miso, tempeh and soy sauce.

Fermented soy milk is to non-fermented soy milk like yogurt is to milk. It is made by inoculating soy milk with good bacteria such as *Lactobacillus acidophilus.* Fermented soy foods have increased amounts of some nutrients such as folate (a B-vitamin) and vitamin K. They also contain increased levels of healthful antioxidants, according to soy researcher Mark Messina, PhD.

Like other legumes, soybeans contain natural compounds that can interfere with the absorption of protein, calcium and zinc. Fermentation reduces the activity of these substances. Fermented soy foods also contain fewer oligosaccharides, sugars that can cause embarrassing gas. While this could be an advantage (especially in social situations), oligosaccharides also act as prebiotics; they feed the beneficial bacteria in our guts, say Messina.

Soybeans contain genistein, a potent isoflavone claimed by some to disrupt fertility and interfere with thyroid and liver functions. In truth, human research has cleared genistein of these threats and found instead that this phytochemical offers protection against osteoporosis and certain types of cancer. Genestein is found in fermented as well as unfermented soy foods.

"The contention that only fermented soy is safe to consume... is simply not true," says Dr. Andrew Weil. He explains that some of the best forms of soy, such as edamame, tofu and soy nuts, are unfermented and are more likely to help than hurt you. "Claims that unfermented soy foods contain toxins that block the action of enzymes needed to digest protein...are misleading," he says. These "trypsin inhibitors" are not just in soy foods; they are found in other vegetables such as cabbage, Brussels sprouts, and beans.

Asians have been using fermented as well as unfermented soy foods for the past 1000 years, says Dr. Messina. In modern Japan, 90 percent of the soy eaten is from tofu, which is not fermented, and miso and natto which is fermented. We can safely enjoy all forms, he assures us.

GOING FOR THE MOLD..ON CHEESE

For the record, I am an Olympic junkie. And while keeping up with our American athletes, I get a bit distracted by the commentators while I'm trying to concentrate on these questions from readers:

Q: "Some people tell me if your cheese gets mold on it, you should throw it all away. Is that true?"

A: I don't know if team USA can recover from this; I mean, it depends on the type of cheese. According to the United States Department of Agriculture Food Safety Inspection Service (USDA-FSIS), cheeses that are high in moisture content can harbor mold below the surface of the food. Best to discard softer cheeses that

Quinn-Essential Nutrition

show any signs of mold including cream cheese, cottage cheese, Neufchatel and any crumbled, shredded or sliced cheese.

Hard and semi-soft cheeses like Cheddar, Colby and Swiss are not easy for mold to penetrate, say food safety experts. We can generally cut away the moldy part of these cheeses and safely eat the rest. Make sure to remove at least one inch around and below the moldy spot, however. And keep the knife away from the mold so it does not contaminate other parts of the cheese.

This guy is a spectacular athlete! Or rather, some molds are harmless, such as the white moldy rind of Brie and Camembert cheeses. Molds used to make cheeses like Roquefort, blue, Gorgonzola, and Stilton are safe to eat as well. Fungus that is not part of the manufacturing process is a problem, however. If you're not sure about any moldy food, toss it, advises the FSIS.

A: "What about mold on bread? I bought bread that had no preservatives and one slice soon had mold on it, so I threw it away. But the other slices didn't, so I ate them. Was this right?

He knows what he has to do to win the gold. I mean, yes, foods without preservatives are apt to mold quicker. And moldy bread should be tossed, says the FSIS. Bread is porous and mold can easily grow beneath its visible surface. After you toss moldy bread, clean the area where it was stored to keep mold from spreading to new loaves.

He has to stay in control through this routine. I mean, here are some ways to stay in control of mold:

- Clean the inside of your refrigerator every few months with a tablespoon of vinegar dissolved into a quart of water. Use a bit of bleach in water to scrub away any signs of black mold that grows along door seals.
- Musty-smelling towels and sponges are signs of growing mold. Wash them in hot soapy water or throw them away.
- Use leftovers within 3 to 4 days..before mold gets a chance to grow. Go team!

Barbara A. Quinn, MS, RD, CDE

IODINE AND YOGURT

Q: "I am 95 percent Californian and 5 percent Missourian which includes not wearing white between Labor Day and Memorial Day and using iodized salt. It occurred to me recently that I have not read anything about iodized salt in decades. Do we need it?"

A: Yes, we need iodine. This essential element is used to make energy-regulating thyroid hormones. Too little iodine causes the thyroid gland to enlarge, a condition called goiter. In infants, a deficiency of iodine can cause mental retardation. Iodine was first added to table salt in 1924 in an effort to curb the incidence of goiter in the United States. It worked; iodine deficiency is now rare in this country. But we don't need to eat more salt to get enough iodine. Just 1/4 teaspoon of iodized salt contains half the iodine we need in a day. Seafood and dairy foods are also good sources of natural iodine.

Q: "Please do not use my name. I am too ashamed of my ignorance. Could you please explain what nutrients a person absorbs when he eats non-fat, plain (no sugar, no fruit) yogurt? What are the negative effects of eating lots of yogurt, like a half pound a day?"

A: Dear anonymous, Eight ounces of non-fat plain yogurt will feed your body about 130 calories of energy with as much protein as 2 ounces of meat, 400 milligrams of calcium (almost half your daily need), plus essential vitamins and minerals. I can think of few negative effects unless you have an allergy to milk or are eating so much yogurt that you skip other important food groups such as vegetables and fruit.

CONSEQUENCES OF FIBER

Q: "I take it the usual person should eat a daily requirement for fiber of 25 to 35 grams. But can one eat too much and how much is too much and if too much is consumed, what are the consequences?"

A: Technically, we need 14 grams of fiber for every 1000 calories we consume. Since most people don't go around calculating how many calories they eat every day, the general recommendation is 25 to 35 grams. Can we eat too much? No "Upper Tolerable Limit" (the amount of fiber above which you may have problems) has been set due to insufficient evidence, according to the Institute of Medicine, the body of experts who make such decisions. One thing is for sure; if you suddenly increase your intake of fiber, you may experience digestive consequences. It's also important to drink plenty of fluids when you eat more fiber.

Q: "Regarding soluble and insoluble fiber, what is an appropriate mix and if one fails on the mix, what are the consequences?"

A: The terms "soluble" and "insoluble" in relation to dietary fiber may be on their way out, since researchers have found that the benefits of fiber have little to do with its solubility. Instead, "viscosity" and "fermentability" seem to better describe the characteristics of dietary fiber, according to a report by the Institutes of Medicine. What is a good mix? Viscous and fermentable fibers from a varied diet of fruits, vegetables, whole grains and beans help control cholesterol, blood sugars and weight.

Q: "A site on the internet states that soluble fiber is found in foods commonly thought of as starches; but soluble fiber differs from starch because the chemical bonds that join its individual sugar units cannot be digested by enzymes in the human body. In other words, soluble fiber has no calories because it passes through the body intact. However, food labels I've read that reflect some dietary fiber seem always to state calories. Could you clarify what this means?"

A: I'd be glad to. Fiber is a carbohydrate that the body cannot digest for energy; thus it does not supply calories, which are units of energy. Sugars and starches are also carbohydrates and they *do* supply energy, or calories, to the body. A slice of whole grain bread, for example, contains starch and fiber. The calories listed on the label come from the starch, not the fiber.

> REFLECTION: *A meta-analysis of prospective studies between 1990 and 2013 concluded, "greater dietary fibre intake is associated with a lower risk of both cardiovascular disease and coronary heart disease." At the time of this writing, the designation for dietary fiber remained unchanged on the Nutrition Facts label.*

SUGAR DEFINITIONS

Dear Ms. Quinn:

Can you define what is meant by "sugar free," "reduced sugar" and "sugar alcohol"? It is quite confusing when shopping for such food items for a pre-diabetic.—Jim

Yes, it can be confusing, Jim. These terms are strictly defined by the US Food and Drug Administration (FDA). "Sugar-free" means the food contains less than 0.5 gram of sugar per serving, a negligible amount. This also applies to the terms "no sugar," "sugarless," or "zero sugar," says the FDA. For example, the "Sugar Free" iced tea I just mixed up with some sliced lemons and mint leaves contains no sugar according to the Nutrition Facts label. Although there is a trivial amount of sugar from added corn syrup solids, this product can still be labeled "Sugar-free" because each serving contains less than a half gram of sugar.

"Reduced Sugar" can be claimed for a food that has at least 25 percent less sugar than its original form. For instance, an 8-ounce cup of Reduced Sugar grape juice contains 18 grams of sugar (about 4 teaspoons) compared to 26 grams (about 6 teaspoons) in regular grape juice.

"No Added Sugars" means no type of sugar has been added to the food. Plain yogurt, without fruit or other sugars, can be labeled "No Added Sugars." But it cannot bear the label, "Sugar-Free" because it contains lactose, a sugar that occurs naturally in milk.

"Sugar alcohols" do not contain alcohol in the intoxicating sense. These sweetening compounds are poorly digested and thus provide about half the calories of table sugar. Examples include xylitol, sorbitol, mannitol, maltitol, and isomalt.

"Low sugar" is a term that the FDA has not defined; therefore it is banned from use on food labels.

Note too, that the term "sugar" has a different definition than "sugars," according to the FDA. "Sugar" specifically means sucrose (table sugar) that is half glucose and half fructose. "Sugars" (plural) includes *all* sugars, including lactose in milk, fructose in fruit, honey and corn syrups. For example, the first ingredient in brownie mix is "sugar" (sucrose), but this product also contains corn syrup. Therefore, the nutrition label informs me there are 16 grams of "sugars" (plural) in one brownie.

MEN ONLY

GUY TO GUY: YOU NEED TO KNOW THIS

"You need to write about this," my guy informed me one Saturday afternoon. "Guys need to know this."

Know about what? I asked as I watched him pull a package of buns and frankfurters out of a grocery bag.

"The hot dog," he said flatly. "It's your Saturday afternoon standard when you're out in the garden."

And your nutritional point? I ask.

"Gardening requires extra nutrition," he said as my eyes rolled toward our daughter. She smiled.

"My hot dogs are just two grams of fat per dog compared to 8 or 9 grams by industry standards," he announced. "And if you smother it with relish and hot sauce, you can't tell the difference. Be sure to cook it in beer, the other half of the beer you didn't drink; that's a guy thing. Cook it a good 10 to 15 minutes at a low boil; that assures a good soft dog for the bun. Just beware of the empty calories in alcohol scenario." Translation: Alcohol contains no redeeming nutritional value except calories that can promote weight gain.

"Another thing guys need to know," he said as he examined a container of chopped tomatoes, onions and peppers. "Skip the dip and go for the salsa. Read the label, guys. Zero fat. It's spicy; it's fresh."

What about the chips? I asked.

"Chips are up to you, of course. And then you have sun tea (tea bags suspended into a large glass jar of water to slowly brew in the sun). Best darn stuff to have while you're in the garden. This is my favorite," he informed me as he pulled out a box of cinnamon spice herb tea. "Get off the caffeine," he said, as I eyed him in amazement.

Next out the bag…"yogurt and granola, God's gift to the gut and colon. Yogurt assists the gut to rebalance itself and the granola cleans out the pipes, or whatever you want to say about that. Make sure, guys, you get yogurt with live and active cultures. Or talk to my buddy Roy, for his homemade yogurt recipe. It's easy."

Next topic: Dessert. "Simple; chop up pears, peaches, mangos, berries. Mix in a little sugar, and maybe a couple taps of allspice. Spoon it over ice cream. It's the best."

And would that be low fat ice cream? I interject.

"Pick your poison. Now about how to make homemade wine…"

Thanks, dear. Maybe next time.

A GUY'S NUTRITION ADVICE TO GIRLS

Young people say it like only young people can. My daughter's college friend, Gary, has definite opinions about the way young women eat (or don't eat) to stay thin.

"I think it's unhealthy," he declared. "Most of the girls I know are worried about what they eat, so they don't eat at all and then they get starving and go eat something that's totally fattening, like cookies or a candy bar or ice cream. I don't understand that."

"My girlfriend is like that," he continued. "She won't eat all day and then she'll go to some fast food place and get tacos or something. And I go, Why are you eating this (stuff)? Why don't you just eat during the day and then you won't be so starving?"

Does she listen? I asked.

"She's starting to…I think."

He then tells me about a female friend in his business class who wants to lose weight. "She started taking those fat-burning diet pills. And I was like, Oh yeah, so it has that ephedra stuff in it? And she's like, 'No, these are ephedra-free but they are supposed to work really good.' And I was all, That's not doing anything for you; it's just all going to come back on you after you stop taking them."

I agreed.

"Those things are bad for you; they can hurt your heart," he said emphatically. Right again. In the process of speeding up heart rate and blood pressure, ephedra, especially in combination with other stimulants like caffeine, has been linked to heart attacks and stroke.

What about guys? I asked. Do they obsess about their weight, too?

"No, and I think that's a stupid double standard," Gary said. "You always see a really hot girl with this big old fat guy and he's all ugly and out of shape. And she's all worried about how her weight is and he's usually telling her that she's gaining weight."

My daughter and I were laughing at this point.

What other advice might a healthy, young college man have for his female friends? I asked.

"Eat smaller meals and add some exercise in there," he advised. "And I don't know if girls think about keeping their calcium (intake) up. I drink milk, 1 percent or fat-free. Girls don't think about that.

Right again. Most young women fail to get their recommended 1000 to 1300 milligrams of calcium in their daily diets. One cup of milk, yogurt, or calcium-fortified soy beverage contains about 300 milligrams.

Any final comments? I asked Gary.

"I see a lot of young people eating bad all the time. But even if you're skinny, it doesn't mean it's not sticking to you on the inside when you get older. A lot of people eat and eat and then they get into their 30's and 40's and all of a sudden they are having all these health problems and they can't figure it out. So I'm trying to bypass all that and try to stay healthy from the get-go now. Because I think in the future, that will be what makes me healthier and not have heart problems and cancer.

Couldn't have said it better myself.

MEN'S HEALTH QUIZ

I love this guy, even when the main ingredient in his "vegetarian" pasta is Italian sausage. I care about his health too, because I want him around for a long time. See how your favorite man does with this quiz:

1. What is the biggest killer of men in the United States? a) auto accidents; b) heart attacks and strokes; c) Viagra. Answer is b. By far, diseased hearts stop more men's lives than any other cause.
2. How often should a man have his blood pressure checked? a) Every year; b) Once a week; c) When he gets up to change the channel. Answer is a). Blood pressure checks should be done at least annually and more often if warranted.
3. How many daily servings of vegetables and fruit does a man need for optimal health? a) two; b) five; c) one can of vegetable juice. Answer is b. At least two pieces of fruit and three helpings of vegetables (especially the bright-colored ones) provide a good dose of fiber, vitamins, minerals and phytochemicals that can help prevent heart disease and certain types of cancer.
4. What nutrients should make up the bulk of a man's diet? a) carbohydrates; b) protein; c) Captain Crunch. Answer: a) Along with protein, carbs supply the energy for building muscles. About half the calories a man ingests each day should come from carbohydrates foods such as vegetables, fruit and whole grains.
5. If your cholesterol test reveals a low LDL number but a high HDL number, you should: a) be dead; b) take a cholesterol lowering medication; c) brag to your friends. Answer: c). A low LDL means your arteries are less prone to fill up with harmful fatty deposits known as plaque. A high HDL means your body is working to keep your arteries clear.

6. What is the best exercise to improve your cholesterol numbers? a) a brisk walk; b) sit-ups; c) pushing away from the table. Answer: All are correct.
7. How many men in the United States have diabetes and don't know it? a) the entire population of Sweetwater, Oklahoma; b) 25,000; c) 2.5 million. Answer: c). According to the *American Diabetes Association*, a third of all men who have diabetes are not aware they have the disease…yet.
8. How much water should a man drink every day if he exercises regularly? a) 6 to 8 cups; b) 10 to 11 cups; c) whatever he can gulp from the water fountain at work. Answer: b). Active men need more fluids than couch jocks. And remember, guys, even mild dehydration can affect performance.

REFLECTION: Statistical data from United States health surveys report that men who have diabetes are becoming more aware about their diagnosis. This is encouraging since early detection and treatment is the key to avoiding health complications.

THE 'MOREL' OF THE STORY

This man is a serious mushroom hunter. Last week, he asked me to raise my right hand and repeat, "I do solemnly promise not to reveal in word, wink, or nod, nor to convey in any way, shape or form, the secret mushroom spot."

Ahh, yes, mushrooms—like the people who hunt for them—are in a class of their own. Neither plant nor animal, mushrooms are the "fruit" of fungus that grows in decaying organic matter such as wood bark and other compost-like material. Nutritionally, they are low in calories; most varieties contain about 20 calories per

Quinn-Essential Nutrition

cup. They also offer a bit of protein (one or two grams per ounce) and fiber. Mushrooms also contain potassium, copper, vitamin D and B-vitamins such as niacin and riboflavin. One Portobello mushroom, for example, has more potassium than a banana, according to the Mushroom Council **www.mushroomcouncil.org**

Depending on where they grow, (I'm sworn to secrecy), mushrooms contain varying amounts of selenium, an antioxidant nutrient that works with vitamin E to gobble up harmful molecules in the body known as free radicals. Research suggests that selenium may be effective to help prevent certain types of cancer, including cancer of the prostate.

Mushrooms are more digestible when they are cooked. Some, like the meatier-tasting Portobello, are great in sandwiches. Mushrooms also add flavor and texture to salads and cooked dishes.

Lest we get overly casual about wild mushrooms, however, it is crucial to know that of the 5000 different types of mushrooms in the United States, about 100 are toxic to humans. A handful—like the deadly *Amanita*—contain one of the deadliest poisons found in nature. Naturalist Barbara Bassett says, "Mushroom hunting is not a hobby for the careless or uninformed. On the other hand, neither is it necessarily the death-defying feat that many people imagine. There are a number of good edible mushrooms that are easy to recognize and hard to confuse with anything dangerously poisonous."

"Morels" of this story:

1. Do your homework before you go out to pick wild mushrooms. Old, bold mushroom hunters are rare. Two good resources are *Mushrooms Demystified* and *All that the Rain Promises and More* by California mycologist, David Arora.
2. Keep it simple. Collect only the mushrooms that are easily identified, such as chanterelle, king bolete, or morel.
3. Seek advice from experts to identify any mushroom you are not absolutely certain about.

4. Be extremely cautious with any mushroom if you have allergies. Even the safest of these foods may cause reactions in susceptible individuals.

No doubt, these mushroomers are fun guys with their fungi. Last week my man cooked up some fresh morels for his 'shrooming fanatical friends. They oohed and aahed and asked the inevitable question: "Where'd you find these?"
I'll never tell.

REFLECTION: Mushrooms continue to gain favor in modern medicine for their anti-inflammatory effects and their role in the treatment of cancer. Studies funded by the National Institutes of Health are currently underway to determine if mushrooms may help protect against breast and prostate cancers in particular.

NUTRITION LESSONS FROM DAD

My research in graduate school sought to determine how children acquire their preferences for certain foods. I asked second-grade elementary school children to tell me about foods they liked or disliked, and why they did or did not like these foods. I was surprised to learn that the biggest influence on little Johnny's or Sarah's "yummy" or "yucky" choices was not mom, but dad. Even when mommy was the main food shopper and cook, daddy had the strongest influence on which foods these kiddos actually preferred to eat.

Our family is a good example. Early on, when they saw their dad almost gag at the sight of zucchini or eggplant, our daughters would follow suit. Years later, dear father had an out-of-body experience with grilled eggplant at one of our favorite restaurants.

He began to grill this vegetable at home while singing its praises. And the girls have followed suit. (I'm still waiting on the zucchini.)

Come to think of it, my dad was probably a major influence in my taste for spicy food. A native of New Mexico, a favorite meal was green chile enchiladas.

Dad also taught me not to be picky about food. He grew up in a large family with 12 siblings; he was always appreciative of most food.

I also learned from my dad to make the best of all eating situations. One of his favorite treats was to pile us into his big Lincoln and drive to Bella Vista, a huge family restaurant on the outskirts of Albuquerque. He always ordered the special, all-you-can-eat fried chicken and fish, coleslaw and fries. Then he'd look around and say, "Isn't this a great place?" After we were more than stuffed, he'd say, "Anyone care for a little spumoni ice cream?"

Pay attention, dads. Your kiddos are watching.

REFLECTION: My dad developed Alzheimer's disease in his later years. Yet, even when he no longer remembered the house where he had presided over so many family dinners, he continued to appreciate every meal we shared with him.

JUST FOR WOMEN

NUTRITION TO PREVENT BIRTH DEFECTS

It almost sounds too good to be true. According to the US Centers for Disease Control and Prevention (CDC), "if all women of childbearing age consumed sufficient folic acid, 50 to 70 percent of birth defects of the brain and spinal cord could be prevented."

Marta and Patrick Lynch know it's true because they have lived it. Their first child was born with spina bifida, or "split spine," in which the spinal column does not completely develop during those first critical weeks of pregnancy.

"Having a child with a birth defect is a devastating experience," says Patrick. Their precious daughter was born with an open wound on her back that was so severe, she lived just three weeks.

"When we learned we had a high risk for having another baby with the same condition, we agreed to participate in a study to see if folic acid (a B-vitamin) could help," Marta explains. Prior to and throughout her next two pregnancies, she started taking a supplement of folic acid. "Subsequently, we had two healthy children. In fact, our son, Evan, just completed a report on this topic in his science class."

How does folic acid prevent these neural tube defects of the brain and spinal cord? By merely doing its job. Among other vital functions, folate (the form found naturally in food) and folic acid (a more stable form used in dietary supplements) is needed by the body for cell division. Like an unfinished house when building

Quinn-Essential Nutrition

supplies run low, too little folate during pregnancy can halt the complete development of a fetus. All women of childbearing age need to understand these basics:

- **Timing is everything.** From the moment of conception to the 29th day of pregnancy, when most women don't even know they are pregnant, folic acid is essential for the complete development of the spinal column. That's why the current recommendation by the US Public Health Service is for *all* women of childbearing age, whether pregnant or not, to consume 400 micrograms of folic acid every day from foods and/or supplements.
- **Eat fortified foods.** Since 1998, the Food and Drug Administration (FDA) has required cereal grains sold in the United States to be fortified with folic acid. Some fortified breakfast cereals, such as *Total*, contain as much folic acid as a vitamin pill.
- **Eat green.** Folate occurs naturally in foliage—from the Latin word "folium" which means "leaf." Good sources include broccoli, spinach, Brussels sprouts, cabbage and asparagus. Legumes like kidney and garbanzo beans are excellent sources as well.

Patrick admits he has developed "a kind of evangelistic attitude" about a woman's need for folate during her childbearing years. "If I see fertile young women, I preach about folic acid," he says. "I don't walk down the street and hand out flyers, but it's something that needs to be told."

Experts agree. According to Dr. Godfrey Oakley, Director of the Birth Defects and Developmental Disabilities division of the CDC., "folic acid is the sleeping giant of preventive medicine."

REFLECTION: Recent studies suggest that adequate folate during pregnancy may also help prevent malformations of the heart and limbs. Folate may also lessen the risk for preeclampsia, a serious condition that can occur during pregnancy. Pregnant women need 600 micrograms of folic acid a day, according to the latest Dietary Reference Intakes established by the National Academy of Sciences, Institute of Medicine (IOM). Non-pregnant adults require 400 micrograms of folate/folic acid a day.

Since 1998, the United States Food and Drug Administration (FDA) has required manufacturers to add folic acid to flour, cornmeal, pasta, rice, bread and other grain products. Are we getting too much? Natural food sources are not a worry, says the IOM. It's not a good idea, however, to take in more than 1000 micrograms of folic acid a day from supplements or fortified foods.

PREGNANCY WEIGHT GAIN GUIDE

I got the phone call soon after my daughter and son-in-law learned the news. "Looks like...I'm pregnant," said daughter. "Of course we are really excited, but I'm not going to get fat like I did the last time; mark my words! Maybe my nutritionist (mom) can help me stay on track."

Why, I would be honored, dear one. Here are a few suggestions to help keep your weight gain within a healthy range.

Use this formula to determine how much weight you should gain during your pregnancy: Multiply your pre-pregnant weight (in pounds) by 703. Divide that total by your height in inches. Divide that total a second time by your height in inches. This number is your BMI (Body Mass Index), upon which your expected weight gain for pregnancy is based.

- Normal (BMI 18.5 to 24.9): If your pre-pregnancy BMI is in this range, you can expect a healthier birth outcome if you gain between 25 to 35 pounds during your pregnancy.

- Overweight (BMI 25 to 29.9): Between 15 to 25 pounds is considered an optimal pregnancy weight gain for women in this weight category.
- Obese (BMI over 30): Women who begin their pregnancies in this BMI range have fewer complications when their weight gain during pregnancy is limited to 11 to 20 pounds.

What's the big deal about gaining weight during pregnancy? Researchers now know that babies in the womb who are bathed in excess fat may be more prone to health problems. They suspect that kids might even be programmed to be obese if mom overeats during her pregnancy. Some studies suggest that high fat diets, even if mom is not overweight, may damage baby's developing organs. In the long run, this could interfere with the ability to regulate food intake and lead to health problems.

How fast, or the rate at which you gain weight during pregnancy, is also important. In general, a woman of normal weight is expected to gain about ten pounds by the middle, or 20th week, of her pregnancy. An overweight woman has better outcomes if she gains no more than five pounds during her first 20 weeks of pregnancy.

Remember to focus on a diet that is "nutrient dense" which means it's loaded with protein, vitamins, minerals, and other essential nutrients. Various types of vegetables, fruit, whole grains, low fat dairy, eggs, lean meats, fish, and poultry can fulfill that goal.

And your nutritionist mom is not the only one who says so. A recent review on this topic by the *National Institutes of Health* concluded, "The quality of daily food intake is the most important and most ignored factor determining pregnancy outcomes."

By the way, dear, these guidelines support the best outcomes for moms as well as babies. You both are important to me.

REFLECTION: Logan Thomas Furman contentedly entered our world on April 21, 2014. His two year-old sister, Frances gently kissed him on the head and declared, "He's so cute!"

Barbara A. Quinn, MS, RD, CDE

AMAZING TRU-BREAST

How do we encourage a woman to breastfeed her infant? This analogy has been adapted several times over the years from various publications:

Tru-Breast is a revolutionary method for infant feeding. Ready in an instant! Less work for mother! Each unit comes with these original features:

- Unique "lull-a-bye" sound unit. As baby nurses, he is lulled to sleep as he hears the familiar soothing heartbeat from his days in the womb.
- Divinely patented formula provides an ideal mix of specialty ingredients to protect baby against illness and infections.
- Matched set of Kwik-Fil holding tanks store milk at a perfect temperature; it's never too hot or too cold. Automatic refill feature supplies 100 percent of baby's nourishment for the first six months of life.
- All *Tru-Breast* units are sturdy and unbreakable, and they are virtually impossible to drop on the floor.
- Baby less hungry than usual? No need to refrigerate leftovers. Units retain milk at a safe temperature which is ready whenever baby is hungry.
- Units are durable and designed to promote healthful development of baby's jaws and gums. Made of long-lasting materials which cannot be accidentally pulled off.
- Units come in pairs and improve with use. Sterile Kwik-Klean nipples give bacteria less chance to grow. They clean easily and do not need to be boiled.
- *Tru-Breast* solves the problem of storing baby's items until the next infant comes along. They are decorative as well as functional. Units are available in a variety of sizes, shapes and colors; and size does not affect their ability to function.
- *Tru-Breast* takes the worry out of traveling with baby. Side-by-side units operate well in warm or cold climates, day or night.

- *Tru-Breast* eliminates the middleman. Direct delivery from the producer to the consumer. Economical dual units cost about 500 calories a day, easing the transition back into pre-pregnancy clothes.
- *Tru-Breast* comes with ingredients that promote healthy gut function and sweeter smelling diapers. Babies fed by this method experience less constipation and diarrhea; and they tend to be less picky about eating as they grow. This may be due to specialized units that extract flavor molecules from mother's food and expose baby to a variety of tastes and smells.

REFLECTION: In 2009, the Academy of Nutrition and Dietetics reaffirmed the position that "exclusive breastfeeding provides optimal nutrition and health protection for the first six months of life, and breastfeeding with complementary foods from six months until at least 12 months of age is the ideal feeding pattern for infants."

Evidence continues to show that infants who are breastfed are better protected from ear infections, intestinal infections and diarrhea, respiratory illness, sudden infant death syndrome, obesity, and high blood pressure. Moms who nurse their babies reduce their risk for breast and ovarian cancer, type 2 diabetes, and postpartum depression.

PRINCESS DIET

I was totally enchanted with the set designed by my friend, Nicole, for a charming play at Carmel's Outdoor Forest Theater. And how sweet that it was nutritionally inspired, a musical fable of *The Princess and the Pea*. Although the princess had issues with a pea, she also had amazing strength and endurance, no doubt from eating well and getting plenty of exercise around the castle.

Princesses and other women are designed differently and have health needs different from men, say experts. Men have stronger, more muscular bodies. Women are softer and endowed with a higher percentage of body fat. Some women have accumulated too much soft tissue, according to the American Heart Association (AHA). Two of every three women in the US are now overweight or obese; and heart disease is the leading cause of death in American women. So without further ado and to protect women from heart disease, the AHA presents these uniquely female guidelines:

1. Do not smoke. Period.
2. Exercise moderately, at least 150 minutes a week. And add another 75 minutes of more vigorous activity.
3. Maintain a healthy body weight, which for most people is a Body Mass Index (BMI) of less than 25.
4. Eat DASH-style, which stands for "Dietary Approaches to Stop Hypertension." This eating pattern offers hope for the princesses in the kingdom to live happily ever after. It includes:
    - Fruit and vegetables, four to five cups each day, including fresh, canned, dried, frozen, raw, cooked and juiced;
    - Fish, six to eight ounces a week, preferably of the darker fattier types like salmon, tuna, and sardines;
    - Whole grains, at least three servings a day. One serving is a slice of whole grain bread or 1/2 cup cooked brown rice, whole grain cereal, or pasta;
    - Nuts, legumes, and seeds, three or more servings a week. Count 1/3 cup of nuts, 2 tablespoons of nut butter, or 1/2 cup of cooked beans or peas count as a serving;
    - Sugar, no more than five tablespoons of added sugar each week, including jam, jelly and any other

sugar-sweetened food or beverage. By the way, those five tablespoons of sugar can be found in just one 16-ounce cup of salted caramel hot chocolate from your favorite coffee shop;
- Alcohol, no more than one drink a day, ladies, which is equivalent to four or five ounces of wine, 12 ounces of beer, or an ounce or so of vodka, whiskey or other spirits;
- Limit foods high in sodium, cholesterol, and saturated fat;
- *Trans*-fats, zero, none, nada. These fats are being phased out of our food supply; and that's good for our princess hearts.

MANAGING GESTATIONAL DIABETES

I was jolted out of bed at 4:45 in the morning. The horses were out of their pens, to places unknown. Fearing they might wander into traffic, I called the sheriff.

"What color are the two horses?" the dispatcher asked.

A sorrel and a bay, I said.

"Ma'am, I don't know horse colors. Are they black, white, yellow...?"

Two brown horses, I said.

Another kind of confusing jolt is finding out you have gestational diabetes, a condition that complicates almost 1 in every 100 pregnancies. Here are some helpful facts:

If you have gestational diabetes (GDM), you did not cause it by eating too much sugar. This condition is the result of hormones released toward the end of pregnancy that work against the body's ability to control blood sugar levels. You are more susceptible to develop GDM if you have diabetes in your family or are overweight.

If you have GDM, your nutritional needs are the same as any other pregnant woman. However, you will need to eat carefully balanced meals and snacks to keep blood sugar levels within a safe range. You will especially need to limit your intake of foods that are high in carbohydrates, sugars and starches in beverages and desserts and those that occur naturally in fruit, grains, and milk. Excess carbohydrates can cause your blood sugar levels to pop up too high. Complications of uncontrolled blood sugars during pregnancy include delivery of a large baby (9 pounds or more) and an increased risk for the infant to develop obesity and type 2 diabetes later in life.

Physical activity is another powerful way to control your blood sugars if you have gestational diabetes. Walking and other gentle exercises are generally recommended unless your doctor has reason to advise against it.

Diet and exercise, and sometimes a medication such as insulin, are the tools that work well to control diabetes during pregnancy. And what a relief it is to bring that little one safely into the world!

(Yes, my horses got home safely that morning, too.)

RECIPE FOR MULTIPLE BUNS IN THE OVEN

So, you're expecting a baby. No, you're expecting two or three babies...at the same time. Multiple births are not that uncommon; some are due to fertility treatments and others because older women are now bearing children. (Twins are more common with advancing age.) Recent data shows a continuous rise in the incidence of twin and triplet births in the United States. As of 2011, one in every 30 births resulted in twins, according to the Center for Disease Control and Prevention (CDC). Triplets currently account for one of every 729 births.

"Multifetal" pregnancies carry some risks. These babies are often born too soon and too small (less than 5.5 pounds), before they have attained optimal growth and development.

What's the best recipe for a double or triple batch of healthy babies? Start with the right ingredients. Bones, brains, and beautiful bodies are molded from nutrients found in food and consumed by mommies-in-waiting. Calories (energy) from the right foods provide fuel to develop these tiny little ones into bright little bundles of joy. From the test kitchen of nutrition research comes this proven recipe for multiple buns in the oven:

1. Blend three or more cups of milk, yogurt, or calcium-fortified soy or rice beverage into each day.
2. To each meal, add protein-rich foods such as eggs, nuts, meat, fish, poultry, Greek yogurt, or beans.
3. Combine with generous servings of whole grain bread, cereal, crackers, rice or pasta;
4. Add four liberal cups of vegetables and fruit and stir well.
5. Sprinkle with small amounts of essential omega-3 fats including alpha linolenic acid (ALA), docosahexaenoic acid (DHA), and eicosapentaenoic acid (EPA). Nutrition chefs say these are vital for optimal development of babies' brains and vision. Find ALA in soybean and canola oils, flaxseed, walnuts, Brussels sprouts, kale, spinach, and salad greens. Look for DHA and EPA in fatty fish such as salmon, tuna, sardines and trout.
6. Divide mixture into three or more portions and consume over the course of each day during pregnancy. Additional prenatal vitamin and mineral supplements can be added as directed by your health care provider.
7. Set timer for 38 to 40 weeks and carefully monitor the growth of the buns in the oven.
8. Use a scale to check the adequacy of your recipe. Weight should rise gradually by four to six pounds over the first 12 weeks of pregnancy. After that, expect a steady gain of approximately 1 to 2 pounds each week.
9. When recipe is fully developed, remove ever so gently. Keep warm and serve immediately to mom and dad.

Barbara A. Quinn, MS, RD, CDE

> REFLECTION: In 2009, pregnancy weight gain recommendations based on a woman's pre-pregnancy weight and body mass index (BMI) were published by the Institutes of Medicine (IOM). A woman with twins who begins her pregnancy at a normal weight should gain 37 to 54 pounds, says the IOM. An overweight woman with twins can safely gain 31 to 50 pounds. And the recommended weight gain for an obese women carrying twins is 25 to 42 pounds.

APPLAUSE FOR MENOPAUSE

My friend Michelle wanted to help me laugh about my impending birthday. So she treated me to a musical play about menopause, what was billed as "the hilarious celebration of women and the change." Very funny.

"Anyone want to buy a hot flash fan?" a woman called to theatre patrons as we settled into our seats. I tried to smile. When the play began, I recognized several familiar tunes from the 60's and 70's, except someone had changed the lyrics. To a well-known Beach Boys melody about California girls, four mature women belted out, "I wish we all could be sane and normal girls!" Another familiar tune about "my guy" now addressed the woes of gaining weight: "Nothing I can do, cuz it sticks like glue, to my thighs... my thighs." Cute.

Menopause is quite literally the permanent "pause" in menstrual periods that happens when a woman is around the age of 50. In polite circles, it's known as "the change." And boy howdy, do we change. Our bodies, our bones and our moods are altered, mostly due to a decline in the hormone estrogen. Some women sail through these changes; others not so well. Here are some ways nutrition may help:

Quinn-Essential Nutrition

- Limit alcohol to no more than one drink a day, ladies. And that "one" drink is a mere 5 ounces (a bit more than a half cup) of wine, 12 ounces of beer (one bottle or can) or a mixed drink made with about an ounce of liquor. Weight gain, a common side effect of menopause, is less likely when we don't overdo empty calories from alcohol.
- Cut back on caffeine. Stimulants found in coffee, tea, sodas, and chocolate can trigger hot flashes, those annoying little power surges caused by estrogen loss.
- Save your bones. Estrogen works with vitamin D to absorb calcium; when estrogen falls, so does bone mass. Menopausal women need 1000 to 1500 milligrams of calcium each day. Boron, a trace mineral found in milk, broccoli, peanuts, raisins and celery, can also help maintain bone mass as well as mental alertness.
- Exercise your brain. Short term memory can be affected by the loss of...what was the name of that hormone again? As estrogen declines, we can keep our brains popping with physical and mental activities. Why not just replace the estrogen we've lost? Many women do...or did, prior to results from the Women's Health Initiative that advised against routine hormone replacement therapy. Pity.
- Get some estrogen from your food. According to the National Institutes of Health (NIH), "phytoestrogens" occur naturally in more than 300 plant foods and herbs. Two main categories are isoflavones in soy foods, garbanzo beans, and legumes, and lignans in flaxseed, bran, legumes, beer and bourbon (really). According to a position paper by the *Academy of Nutrition and Dietetics*, soy foods may relieve hot flashes and other symptoms of diminished estrogen. Not everyone advocates to use of isolated soy isoflavone supplements, however, due to a lingering question of whether these substances may increase the risk for breast cancer in some women. Best to get natural phytoestrogens in food.

- Age gracefully. Interestingly, in cultures such as Asia where age and wisdom are valued more than youth and beauty, the icky symptoms of menopause are rare. These cultures also have a higher lifetime intake of soy-based foods.

REFLECTION: Hot flashes and other irritating symptoms of menopause have caused some women to seek relief from certain herbal products. Registered dietitian Judith Thalheimer discussed some of these in a 2013 article in Today's Dietitian:

Soy isoflavone extracts are substances in plants that act as weak estrogens and may help ease hot flashes in doses of 35 to 120 milligrams daily. Genistein may be particularly helpful at a dose of 15 milligrams per day, according to the Natural Medicines Comprehensive Database. CAUTION: Although naturally occurring phytoestrogens in soy and other foods have been found to be safe and even beneficial for women with a history of breast cancer, concentrated doses from supplements are probably not a good idea for any woman at risk for breast cancer.

Black cohosh has shown some benefit in the treatment of hot flashes, according to limited evidence, says Thalheimer. Some side effects have been reported, including stomach upset and headaches. Liver damage has also been reported in some cases.

Red clover is a concentrated source of phytoestrogens. Women with a history of breast cancer are advised to avoid this herb or use it with caution.

DRINK TO HEALTH

REASONS TO HAVE A CUP OF TEA

*There is no trouble so great or grave
that cannot be much diminished by a nice cup of tea.*
—Bernard-Paul Heroux, Basque philosopher

What is it about a cup of hot tea that is so...soothing? I personally think it's the warmth that emanates from pretty tea cups. But scientists credit a host of natural compounds in tea for its beneficial effects.

Interesting, all tea comes from the same plant: *Camellia sinensis*. Over the centuries, according to the USDA Agricultural Research Service, this plant formed chemicals called "polyphenols" to protect itself from the elements. Part of a larger family called "flavonoids," these substances are health promoting antioxidants. When tea leaves are processed into the various forms of tea, their flavonoid content changes, say researchers. Green tea, for example, contains more simple antioxidant flavonoids, while black tea contains more complex varieties.

Green, black and oolong teas belong to the same *C. sinensis* plant; they are just processed differently. Green tea is minimally fermented, which is the process of exposing the leaves to air and letting them dry. Black tea is fermented to the greatest extent. And the fermentation of oolong tea is somewhere in the middle. Beside the fact that tea contains zero calories and soothes your soul, here are other compelling reasons to enjoy a cup of tea:

- Curb food cravings. "Afternoon tea" was supposedly started by the 7th Duchess of Bedford (England) to keep her hunger pangs at bay between lunch and dinner. And from personal experience, I find a cup of tea curbs the search for food in those munch-prone evening hours.
- Lower cholesterol. Some studies have shown that tea drinking can help to lower "bad" LDL cholesterol levels. Powerful antioxidant substances in tea are believed to be the reason.
- Fight infections. Several compounds have been found in black and green teas that actually work like antibiotics to fight off the bad bugs that make us sick.
- Prevent halitosis (bad breath). Swishing your mouth with tea can suppress foul mouth odor, say experts. Researchers at the University of Illinois say it's the polyphenols in tea that inhibit the growth of bacteria in the mouth.

What about herbal teas? While not the official *Camellia sinensis* tea, infusions from the leaves of other plants may have their own benefits, according to scientists at Tufts University. Chamomile and peppermint teas, for example, appear to have infection fighting capabilities. Peppermint tea is rich in antioxidants that inhibit the growth of cancer cells. And a clinical trial at Tufts found that drinking three cups of hibiscus tea every day for six weeks helped lower blood pressure in adult volunteers.

Want to make a perfect cup of tea? Here are the key steps, according to Cindy Bigelow, whose grandmother invented Constant Comment® tea:

Start with cold fresh water every time, not the leftover in your tea kettle. "It's the oxygen in the water that opens up the tea leaf for full flavor extraction," says Bigelow.

For black and oolong teas, bring the water to a rolling boil and then pour over leaves or tea bag. Steep for one or two minutes. For more delicate green teas, use water that has just begun to boil. Steep for three to four minutes.

Do not, do not squeeze your teabag into your tea! says Bigelow. This releases bitter tannins that destroy flavor.

Lastly, as the adage goes, "Remember the tea kettle; it is always up to its neck in water, yet it still sings!"

REFLECTION: Regular or Decaf? Both types of tea contain flavonoids, potent antioxidant substances that can inactivate out of control oxygen molecules and offer some protection against heart disease and certain cancers. Decaffeinated tea generally contains fewer flavonoids.

Hot or Iced? Brewed tea at any temperature retains its health benefits, say experts. And if it's brewed, it has superior antioxidant properties to instant or bottled tea.

In 2012, the 5th International Scientific Symposium on Tea & Human Health convened in Washington, DC to review more than 5,600 recent studies on tea. Among the findings:

- *Green tea (and the caffeine it contains) helps enhance the body's ability to burn calories and fat for energy;*
- *As little as one cup of black tea per day may help reduce blood pressure and counter the adverse effect of a high fat meal on blood vessels;*
- *Flavanols in green tea can help strengthen bones when accompanied by weight-bearing exercise;*
- *Drink two to three cups of black tea while on the job; it can improve mental sharpness and your ability to focus;*
- *Tea contains "bioactive compounds" that appear to impact every cell in the body in a positive way, says Jeffrey Blumberg, PhD, Director of the Antioxidants Research Laboratory, Jean Mayer USDA Human Nutrition Research Center on Aging at Tufts University in Boston. "An overwhelming body of research from around the world indicates that drinking at least a cup of green, black, white or oolong tea a day can significantly enhance human health."*

Barbara A. Quinn, MS, RD, CDE

LEARNING ABOUT CAFFEINE

Among other things, I learned to drink coffee when I was in college...from a cute cowboy named Carl. Carl liked coffee and I didn't. So he'd fix me a cup loaded with cream and sugar and then I *really* didn't like it.

Eventually, the time came when I needed to study for an exam late into the night. It was then that I decided, if I was going to drink coffee, I'd drink it black. And so I did, until years later when I fell in love with good coffee and real cream; but that's another story.

Caffeine is the active ingredient in coffee that can raise blood pressure in susceptible people. And if you drink a cup of black coffee an hour before a high carbohydrate meal, it could send your blood sugar levels up higher than normal, according to some research. Moderate coffee drinking, 3 cups or 300 milligrams of caffeine a day, has not been linked to adverse health effects, however. In fact, large prospective studies in several countries including the United States found that coffee consumption is associated with a lower risk for type 2 diabetes.

A study in France found an association between women who consumed at least three cups of coffee a day and a slower rate of decline in cognitive thinking. That got my attention.

And perhaps the best argument for a cup of coffee comes from this piece that appeared in our hospital auxiliary newsletter:

"A philosophy professor stood in front of his class and held up a large mayonnaise jar. Without speaking, he proceeded to fill the jar with golf balls. He then asked the students, 'Is the jar full?'

They agreed that it was. He then began to pour pebbles into the jar that settled into spaces between the golf balls.

'Is the jar full now?' he asked.

Again the students agreed that it was. The professor then commenced to pour sand into the jar, where it filled the remaining spaces between the balls and the pebbles. Once again the class agreed that now the jar was truly full. The instructor then produced two cups of coffee and filled the jar to the brim.

'This jar,' he explained, 'represents your life. The golf balls are the important things—your family and friends, your health and your passions. If you lost everything but these, your life would still be full. The pebbles are other meaningful things in your life—your job, your house, your car. The sand is everything else...the small stuff.

'If you put sand into the jar first,' he continued, 'there is no room for the pebbles or golf balls. Same goes for life. If you spend all your time and energy on the small stuff, you will never have time for the things that are really important. Make room for the important things in your life. The rest is just sand.'

'What about the coffee?' one student asked.

The professor smiled and said, 'It shows that no matter how full your life may seem, there is always room for a cup or two of coffee with a friend."

REFLECTION: How is it that plain coffee can increase blood sugar levels in some people? It's probably the caffeine which stimulates the nervous system, says the American Diabetes Association. If you have diabetes, you may want to check your blood sugars after drinking coffee to see if it affects you in this way. Sudden withdrawal from caffeine can affect you big time, according to a study of people who considered themselves moderate coffee drinkers. In the first two days without caffeine, volunteers described being extremely fatigued and unable to concentrate. Some of them even resorted to pain medication, thinking they had the flu.

Caffeine stimulates the mental processing part of the brain; it helps us be more alert although not necessarily smarter. Athletes have found that caffeine can enhance physical endurance. Caffeine is even added to some pain medications to improve their effectiveness.

Previous studies pointed to caffeine as a risk factor for osteoporosis. Yet researchers now say that this negative effect may have been overstated. How? New evidence points to flavonoids and polyphenols in caffeinated beverages like coffee and tea that may actually enhance bone health.

On the negative side, excess caffeine can irritate the lining of the stomach and worsen diarrhea, especially if you already have a sensitive stomach. Caffeine also acts like a diuretic; it flushes water out of your system. When this happens, nutrients that are soluble in water such as B-vitamins and vitamin C are washed away as well.

Caffeine crosses the placenta during pregnancy, meaning baby gets a jolt from mom's morning java. Caffeine can show up in breast milk within an hour after ingestion, although the amount may not be significant. One study calculated if mom drinks five ounces of coffee (or about 100 milligrams of caffeine), her nursing baby will be exposed to less than three milligrams of caffeine over the next 24 hours.

Some evidence suggests that drinking more than four cups of coffee a day during pregnancy is associated with lower birth weights. No good evidence to date, however, has shown that caffeine intake is related to birth defects, according to reports by the National Institutes of Health.

What is a safe dose of caffeine? Most experts recommend not more than 200 to 300 milligrams a day; that's two or three dainty (5-ounce) coffee cups. If you guzzle from a mug, better measure how much it holds. One measuring cup (8 ounces) of coffee holds about 200 milligrams of caffeine, enough for some folks to feel caffeine's "pharmacological" effects.

If you are a tea drinker, remember that the longer it brews, the more caffeine it contains. An 8-ounce cup of tea brewed for one minute contains just 40 milligrams of caffeine. Steep it for five minutes and the caffeine level goes up to 60 milligrams. Hot cocoa contains a small amount of caffeine, but you would have to drink ten cups to get the same amount of caffeine found in one cup of coffee.

COFFEE PERKS

When I emailed a friend that I was at a meeting of the Hawaii Coffee Association, he replied, "A nutritionist at a coffee convention? Just curious."

I was curious, too. But hey, where else do you get 100 percent Kona coffee breaks? And speakers in Hawaiian shirts? I was alert and ready to learn.

For starters, I learned that Hawaii is the only coffee producing state in America. Coffee trees love the dense sunshine, plentiful rain, and rich volcanic soil of these islands. And growers work hard to produce healthy coffee plants that produce good-tasting coffee; more than 30 varieties are grown in Kona alone. Coffee labeled "100% Kona coffee" is harvested exclusively from beans grown in this region.

Besides the fact that much of the world does not function in the morning without it, does coffee contain any redeeming health value? Why, yes, it does, say experts. A recent study at John Hopkins University found that 200 milligrams of caffeine (what we might get in 8 to 12 ounces of brewed coffee) enhanced the ability of study participants to remember details.

But coffee is more than just a vehicle for caffeine, say researchers at Harvard University. Our morning brew embodies hundreds of different compounds, including protective antioxidant substances. Coffee also supplies the minerals magnesium and chromium, which the body uses with the hormone insulin to regulate blood sugar levels. In fact, recent studies report an association between higher coffee intakes and lower risks for type 2 diabetes.

Still, it's not a good idea for everyone to down a carafe of coffee every morning. Because the caffeine in coffee crosses the placenta to growing babies, pregnant women are advised to limit coffee intake to no more than one or two cups a day. If you have high blood pressure, you should carefully monitor how caffeine may affect you. And according to Harvard researchers, "If you're drinking so much coffee that you get tremors, have sleeping problems, or feel stressed and uncomfortable, then obviously you're drinking too much coffee."

I also learned how "cupping" experts use a precise scoring method to rate speciality coffees. Good coffee might be described as rich-bodied with mild acidity, clean, or balanced. Bad coffee might taste dusty, dirty, or "like hot electrical components." Interesting too, that inferior coffee gets worse as it cools. Good coffee gets better.

Kona coffee beans are delicate, explains Tommy Greenwell, a fourth generation coffee farmer at Greenwell Farms in the heart of Kona. Most coffee from this region tastes best at medium roast, not dark, he explains. Tommy's favorite variety? "Jeni K," which he named after his wife.

Why is Kona coffee so pricey? Mostly because of labor costs, says Greenwell's chief financial officer, Steve Hicks. Each individual coffee "cherry," the red ripe fruit of the coffee tree that produces a coffee bean, is hand-picked in this coffee-growing region of the world.

Store your precious beans in airtight containers away from direct light and heat, and never put coffee in the refrigerator, advises Peggy, our enthusiastic tour guide at Greenwell Farms. Moisture causes coffee to deteriorate. She also advises coffee lovers to only buy what you will use within a week or two. Ground coffee, in particular, quickly loses quality and flavor if stored too long. And, she adds, when you drink good coffee, you don't need cream or sugar.

After my visit to the big island of Hawaii, I agree with these coffee growers: "To drink is human. To drink Kona coffee is divine." Mahalo and aloha.

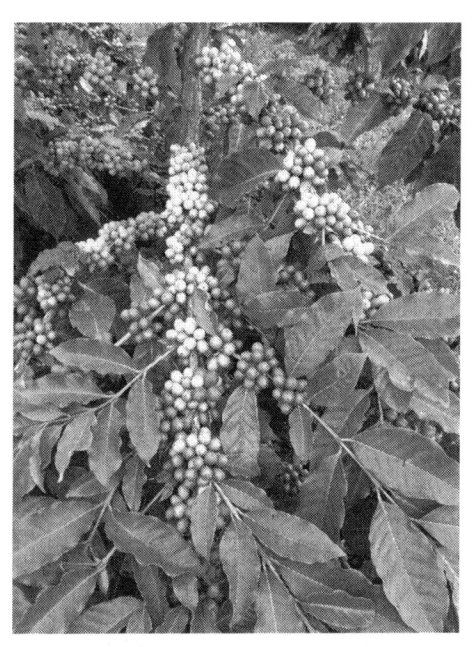

Coffee tree at Greenwell Farms, Kona Hawaii

BENEFITS AND RISKS OF KOMBUCHA TEA

Sweeten black tea with sugar. Add yeast and friendly bacteria cultures. Allow to ferment for several days. What do you get? Kombucha (Kom-BOO-cha) tea, a fermented beverage consumed for its reported health benefits. Here are a few reports from recent studies:

An article in the *Journal of Science of Food and Agriculture* notes that Kombucha tea contains "potential hepato-protective agents." Translation: Some substances in Kombucha could possibly be good for the liver, the body's main detox unit.

Biochemists reporting in the journal of *Food Research International* observed that Kombucha interfered with enzymes that digest starch. Is that good? Undigested starch might result in lower blood sugar levels for people with diabetes, scientists theorize. Undigested starch may also contribute to gas, I would theorize.

Researchers in Switzerland found that Kombucha tea had "antimicrobial activity," the ability to fight off infections from bacteria, yeast, and other microorganisms. Some of the bacterial cultures in this tea might also deter *Candida,* a microbe that can cause yeast infections, say experts.

There's just one problem. While studies suggest potential benefits to consuming Kombucha tea, none to date have actually tested it on humans. Rodents, yes; one study tested unfermented black tea and fermented Kombucha tea on rats with diabetes (really). Both these beverages possessed healthful antioxidant properties, these scientists reported; yet they concluded that Kombucha tea had more beneficial properties than black tea.

Since most of us are not rats with diabetes, we should heed some safety concerns that have surfaced when humans drink this fermented tea. The US Food and Drug Administration (FDA) has received reports of harm related to Kombucha, including a rare but fatal condition called "lactic acidosis." For this reason, they tell us to "use caution when making and drinking this tea."

Other concerns come from the American Cancer Society (ACS). Several types of yeast and bacteria can grow when brewing Kombucha, says the ACS. And because cultures and preparation methods vary, this tea may contain contaminants such as molds and fungi that can cause illness. "Since the potential health risks of Kombucha tea are unknown, anyone with an immune deficiency or any other medical condition should consult a physician before drinking the tea," advises the ACS. They also advise against the use of Kombucha by pregnant or breastfeeding women.

WINE AND THE FRENCH PARADOX

It was 1991 when *60 Minutes* television reporter Morley Safer used "The French Paradox" to describe how the wine drinking French eat a high fat diet and yet have a very low rate of heart disease. Numerous explanations for this apparent contradiction followed. One that I found particularly intriguing was presented by registered dietitian Elaine Mackey, at a meeting of the California Dietetic Association. At the time, Mackey was the Executive Director of the Napa Valley Vintner's Association:

Similar to the typical American diet, the French consume between 34 to 37 percent of their daily calories from fat, said Mackey. Yet the rate of heart disease in France is 40 percent less than that of the United States. In fact, France has the second lowest rate of heart disease in the world. What gives?

Wine may be part of the influence, Mackey suggested. Research shows that moderate drinkers have a 20 to 40 percent lower risk of cardiovascular (heart-related) deaths when compared to people who abstain or those who are heavy drinkers. "Moderate" in this context means no more than four to eight ounces of wine per day, with women at the lower range due to gender differences in how we metabolize alcohol.

Researchers have found close to a hundred different compounds in wine that may exert health benefits. Known chemically as "phenols," these natural substances impart characteristic color, flavor, aroma and other complexities to wine, said Mackey. Some phenols have been found to increase the "good" HDL cholesterol and lower the "bad" LDL cholesterol levels in the blood. Others keep blood platelets from clumping together which could help prevent heart attacks. Many of these favorable compounds increase during the fermentation process of wine-making, Mackey explained.

Consider too, *how* the French eat compared to Americans. Their heaviest meal is typically early in the day, before they go to work; as evening approaches, they eat more lightly. The French tend to enjoy leisurely meals, and more often they include wine. Research suggests that food with wine and relaxed conversation can play a critical role in reducing stress and the risk for disease.

In contrast, we Americans are famous for fast grab-n-go food. We eat snacks three times more often than the French; and we tend to consume our heaviest meal in the evening. Interesting too, that while we slam down French fries, our French friends enjoy more fruit and vegetables. Definitely food for thought.

Barbara A. Quinn, MS, RD, CDE

REFLECTION: A 2012 study in the American Journal of Clinical Nutrition found that people who drank two glasses of dry red wine per day had higher levels of beneficial bacteria and lower levels of pathogenic bad bacteria in their gut. Healthy gut flora helps enhance digestion, immunity, metabolism, and skin health, say these experts.

Another report in the August 2013 issue of Environmental Nutrition clarified that grape juice and non-alcoholic red wine offer health advantages that are similar to red wine. Experts credit flavonoids in these beverages for their ability to fend off the oxidation of "lousy" LDL cholesterol in the blood. One particular family of flavonoids called anthocyanins, may actually be better absorbed from grape juice than wine, experts report.

Red wine has a boost over grape juice when it comes to resveratrol, the compound that gives grapes their red color and is believed to exert some protection to the arteries. Because fermentation extracts resveratrol from the skins of grapes, red wine contributes more of this substance than unfermented grape juice.

Too much of a good thing is still not good, however. In 2014, researchers from Oregon Health & Science University and the University of Colorado-Denver were looking to identify the benefits of a dietary supplement that contained resveratrol. When they fed this supplement to pregnant monkeys, they were surprised to find that the offspring of these animals developed abnormalities of the pancreas, the organ that controls blood glucose levels. This concern is real enough to advise pregnant women not to take supplements of resveratrol.

As for excessive alcohol intake, read on...

HOW ALCOHOL AFFECTS NUTRITION

My grandfather used to say that "too much of anything is not good for you." Yet a person with an addiction may find it impossible to moderate his or her habit. In addition to other problems, excessive drinking creates major nutrient deficits which profoundly affect the function of a drinker's body and mind.

Alcohol is a powerful solvent; it can rapidly penetrate and dissolve the structures of living cells. That's why it's used as a disinfectant; it destroys bacterial cells. Unfortunately, when a form of alcohol known as ethanol is consumed in large doses, it also destroys brain cells.

Nutritionally, alcohol is in a league of its own. Unlike carbohydrates, fats and proteins that take time to be broken down (digested) before they enter the bloodstream, alcohol is swept into the blood as soon as it hits the stomach. Treated as a toxin by the body, the processing of other nutrients is stopped so the liver can literally get alcohol out of its system. For example, alcohol dehydrogenase, an enzyme in the liver, can break down about one alcoholic drink per hour. If the liver becomes overwhelmed with alcohol, the processing of fuels, known as fatty acids, get put on hold. A stockpile of fatty acids in the liver causes a serious condition called "fatty liver." Just one night of heavy drinking can cause fat to accumulate in the liver, according to some studies.

In nutrition circles, excess alcohol is never a welcome guest; it robs the body of key nutrients. For example, an alcohol-burdened liver cannot activate vitamin D as it normally does. This may explain, in part, how excess alcohol causes bones to weaken. Too much alcohol also causes the body to lose folate, a B-vitamin essential for the production of rapidly dividing cells. Our intestinal tracts are lined with such cells. So when folate is depleted, our ability to digest and absorb nutrients is severely hampered.

An alcohol-slogged body loses water and valuable minerals that regulate fluid in and out of cells. Heavy drinking also interferes with the processing of protein, even when the drinker eats a balanced diet. Alcohol provides "empty" calories, those with no nutritional value. And the body tends to store excess alcohol calories around the middle, where this appropriately named "beer belly" becomes a risk factor for heart disease and diabetes.

The good news? Liver cells can regenerate and recover when alcohol intake is stopped, say experts. If heavy drinking continues, however, even the best diet cannot overcome the ultimate damage.

REFLECTION: Excess alcohol intake is now a leading cause of premature deaths in our country, according to the Centers for Disease Control and Prevention (CDC). Alcohol abuse accounts for one of every ten deaths among working-age adults in the United States.

NUTRITION HUMOR

APRIL FOOLS

Mr. Johnson was terribly overweight, so his doctor put him on a diet. "I want you to eat regularly for two days," he instructed. "Then skip a day and repeat this procedure for two weeks. By your next appointment, you should have lost at least five pounds."

After two weeks, Mr. Johnson returned and his doctor was shocked that he had dropped more than 20 pounds. "This is amazing!" the doctor exclaimed. "You did this by following my instructions?"

The slimmed-down Mr. Johnson nodded. "I'll tell you though, that third day, I thought I was going to drop dead."

"From hunger?" asked the doctor.

"No," replied Mr. Johnson, "from skipping."

* * *

An elderly couple had been in excellent health for many years because of the wife's insistence on a strict regimen of healthful food and daily exercise. One day, they died suddenly in a car accident.

When they reached the pearly gates, St. Peter showed them to their new home, a beautiful mansion with a swimming pool and jacuzzi. The old man asked how much all this would cost.

St Peter smiled and said, "It's free. This is Heaven." He then showed them a freshly groomed golf course right out their back door, with unlimited golfing privileges.

"What are the green fees?" the old man asked.

"You play for free," Peter replied. "This is Heaven." He then ushered them to a lavish buffet in the club house with cuisines from around the world.

"How much to eat here?" the man inquired.

"Don't you understand yet?" said St. Peter. "This is Heaven. All of it is free!"

"Where is the low fat, low calorie food?" asked the wife.

"That's the best part of all," said Peter. "You can eat whatever you like and you never get fat and you never get sick. This is Heaven."

At that, the old man flew into a fit of anger, throwing his hat on the ground and stomping it. His surprised wife asked him what was wrong.

"This is all your fault!" he shrieked. "If it weren't for your blasted bran muffins, I could have been here ten years ago!"

CORNY FOOD JOKES

A man goes to his dentist because something is wrong with his mouth. After a brief examination, the dentist exclaims, "Wow! That plate I installed in your mouth six months ago is almost completely corroded! What on earth have you been eating?"

"Well," the man thought, "about four months ago, my wife made me some asparagus with Hollandaise sauce. And doc, I'm talkin' delicious! I've been putting it on everything—meat, fish, toast, vegetables—you name it!"

"That's probably it," said the dentist. "Hollandaise sauce is made with lemon juice, which is acidic and highly corrosive. I'll have to install a new plate in your mouth, but made out of chrome this time."

"Chrome?" the man asked. "Why chrome?"

"Sir, everyone knows...there's no plate like chrome for the Hollandaise!"

* * *

Quinn-Essential Nutrition

Onntha Cobb was crowned Corn County's new Queen last week. A member of a local family, Onntha is the daughter of a retired kernel. Those who watched the competition say she creamed the other contestants. Cobb, a rather husky girl, wore a yellow silk dress and all the judges---including local celebrities Pop and Caramel Corn---agreed she was very sweet. When presented with a big bushel of flowers, Cobb just smiled and said, "Shucks."

Asked how it felt to be canned by the winner, the first runner-up gave a frozen smile and replied, "I wish I had been picked." Cobb says she is proud of her roots and plans to stalk out a career in her chosen field.

DOUGHBOY AND OTHER FAVORITES

A customer walks into a restaurant and notices a large sign on the wall that says, "$500 if we fail to fill your order."

When the waitress arrives, the man orders elephant tail on rye. She calmly writes it down and walks into the kitchen. Almost immediately the customer hears an explosion of voices from the staff. The restaurant owner then storms out to the customer's table and slaps down five $100 bills.

"You got me this time, buddy," he says, "but I want you to know... that's the first time in 10 years we've been out of rye bread."

* * *

Pillsbury Doughboy, veteran of the baking industry, died last week of a severe yeast infection and complications from repeated pokes in the belly. He was 76.

Buried in a lightly greased coffin, Doughboy's graveside was piled high with flours. Dozens of celebrities turned out for his service, including Mrs. Butterworth, Hungry Jack, and Betty Crocker. Longtime friend, Aunt Jemima, delivered the eulogy, describing Doughboy as someone who "never knew how much he was kneaded."

Barbara A. Quinn, MS, RD, CDE

Despite being flaky at times, Doughboy rose quickly in his profession. His life however, was filled with turnovers. Not considered a very smart cookie, he wasted much of his dough on half-baked schemes. He became hardened and crusty in his later years although many still considered him a roll model.

Doughboy was preceded in death by his famous and flamboyant father, Pop Tart. He is survived by his wife, Play Dough, two children, John and Jane Dough, and a bun in the oven. The funeral was held in the afternoon at 350 for about 20 minutes.

* * *

Sally was driving home from one of her business trips in Northern Arizona when she saw an elderly Navajo woman walking along the side of the road. Since the trip was a long one, Sally stopped the car and asked the older woman if she would like a ride. With a silent nod of thanks, the woman got into the vehicle.

Resuming her journey, Sally tried in vain to make small talk with her passenger. The old woman remained silent, looking intently at everything she saw. Studying the interior of the car, the woman noticed a paper bag on the seat next to Sally.

"What's in the bag?" asked the old woman.

Sally looked down at the brown bag and said, "It's a bottle of wine. I got it for my husband."

The Navajo woman was silent for another moment or two. Then, speaking with the quiet wisdom of an elder, she said: "Good trade."

FUN WITH POTATOES

More potassium per serving than a banana, a good source of vitamin C, and because they spend their life under the soil, potatoes are rich in minerals such as calcium, iron and zinc. In their natural state, these spuds contain no fat or cholesterol and a miniscule amount of sodium. They provide fiber and necessary carbohydrates to fuel the brain and muscles.

Quinn-Essential Nutrition

But oh, how we mistreat these simple spuds. We peel 'em and fry 'em in fat and drench them with salt. And then we totally reject them, forgetting their original goodness.

This "potato" story is adapted from one that appeared in *Capsules,* the monthly newsletter of The Auxiliary at the Community Hospital of the Monterey Peninsula:

Mr. and Mrs. Potato Head had eyes for each other and soon sprouted a sweet little potato named Yam. Yam grew up to be quite a dish and was loved by many.

Not wishing to keep her underground, Mr. and Mrs. Potato Head helped Yam dig into the facts of life. They warned her not to go out half-baked and get smashed or she would be labeled a hot potato and end up with a bunch of tater tots.

Yam told them not to worry; that no spud would get her into the sack and make her a rotten potato! On the other hand, she did not want to stay home and become a couch potato.

Wishing to be a shoestring, Yam parted company with her friends, Au Gratin and Hash Brown. She mashed together what she had and went off to Europe. Mr. and Mrs. Potato warned her not to get into hot water with Irish potatoes and not to be enticed by French fries. Alas, Yam found that most of the tubers she met were twice-baked. When she was done, she returned home.

Mr. and Mrs. Potato then sent Yam to a university in Idaho with hopes that she might meet a high class Yukon Gold and soon be in the chips. One day she announced she was going to marry a high-starched newscaster. This news made Mr. and Mrs. Potato boil. They told Yam there was no way she could butter them up; they would not allow this marriage.

With tears in her eyes, Yam asked, "Why?"

"Because," they said, "he is just a common tater!"

Barbara A. Quinn, MS, RD, CDE

PROOF LAUGHTER IS GOOD FOR YOUR HEALTH

Once upon a time, Old King Cole issued an order to his cooks. "From now on," he decreed, "chopped cabbage must be mixed with mayonnaise." And to this day, this decree has come to be known as "Cole's Law."

* * *

A man sits down at a bar. "Nice tie!" he hears a voice say to him. He looks around but sees no one.

He takes a sip of his beer and hears another voice say, "Great haircut!" He turns and looks behind him and still sees no one. Shaking his head, he turns back to his drink.

"Nice suit!" comes a voice that seems to be nearby.

"Bartender!" he yells. "Who keeps talking to me?"

"Oh, that," says the bartender. "Those are the complimentary peanuts."

* * *

A man goes to his doctor. "You've got to help me, Doc!" he begs. "Something that looks like a lettuce leaf is growing out of my ear." The doctor examines the man, steps back and looks very concerned.

"What is it?" the man asks. "Is it serious?"

"I'm afraid," the doctor says, "it's just the tip of the iceberg."

* * *

Conclusions from nutrition research studies:

The Japanese eat very little fat and suffer fewer heart attacks than the British or Americans.

The French eat a lot of fat and also suffer fewer heart attacks than the British or Americans.

The Japanese drink very little red wine and suffer fewer heart attacks than the British or Americans.

The Italians drink excessive amounts of red wine and also suffer fewer heart attacks than the British or Americans.

Conclusion: Eat and drink what you like. It's speaking English that kills you.

* * *

A man walks into the emergency room with a carrot poking out of one eye. A zucchini is shoved up his nose. A banana is pushed into his ear. The doctor examines him and says, "Nurse! This man hasn't been eating properly!"

* * *

A cannibal says to his friend, *"I don't like my mother-in-law." His friend replies, "That's ok, just eat the noodles."*

* * *

Kevin walks into a doctor's office and the receptionist asks him what he has. He says, "Shingles." So she writes down his name, address, medical insurance number and tells him to have a seat.

Fifteen minutes later, a nurse's aide comes out and asks Kevin what he has. He says, "Shingles." So she measures his height and weight, takes a complete medical history and tells Kevin to wait in the examining room.

A half hour later a nurse comes in and asks Kevin what he has. He says, "Shingles." So the nurse takes his blood pressure, draws a blood sample, and tells him to take off his clothes and wait for the doctor.

An hour later the doctor comes in and finds Kevin sitting patiently in his underwear. He asks Kevin what he has. Kevin says, "Shingles."

"Where?" the doctor asks. Kevin says, "Outside on the truck. Where do you want me to unload 'em?"

* * *

A horse walks into a bar. The bartender says, "Hey."
The horse says, "You read my mind, buddy."

* * *

A man is seated at a restaurant. He studies the menu for a few minutes and asks the waiter, "How do you prepare your chicken?"

The waiter looks at him and says, "We tell them straight up they're not going to make it."

* * *

A rabbi and a priest meet at their town's annual picnic. Old friends, they begin their usual banter.

"This baked ham is really delicious," the priest teases the rabbi. "You really ought to try it. I know it's against your religion, but I can't understand why such a wonderful food should be forbidden! You don't know what you're missing. You just haven't lived until you've tried Mrs. Hall's prized ham. Tell me, Rabbi, when will you break down and try it?"

The rabbi smiles at the priest and grins, "At your wedding."

REFERENCES AND RESOURCES

Academy of Nutrition and Dietetics, www.eatright.org

Alliance for Food and Farming, www.safefruitsandvegetables.com

American Cancer Society, www.cancer.org

American Diabetes Association (ADA), www.diabetes.org

American Egg Board, www.aeb.org

American Institute of Cancer Research, www.aicr.org

Anorexia nervosa, *Diagnostic and Statistical Manual of Mental Disorders* (5th ed.), American Psychiatric Association, 2013.

Biotechnology, www.ucbiotech.org

Bone health, *Journal of the Academy of Nutrition and Dietetics,* January 2014; 114:1, 72-85; *Nutrition Research Reviews,* June 2007; 20(1): 89-105.

Breakfast eating and weight change in a 5-year prospective analysis of adolescents: Project EAT (Eating Among Teens). *Pediatrics* 2008;121:638-645

Breakfast habits, nutritional status, body weight, and academic performance in children and adolescents, *Journal of the American Dietetic Association,* 2005;105: 743-760

Cancer risks and benefits associated with a potential increased consumption of fruits and vegetables, *Food and Chemical Toxicology,* Vol 50, Issue 12, December 2012, pp. 4421-4427.

Celiac Disease, National Foundation for Celiac Awareness, http://www.celiaccentral.org/celiac-disease/facts-and-figures/

Chile, Gastro-protection induced by capsaicin in healthy human subjects, Gyula Mózsik, János Szolcsányi, István Rácz, *World Journal of Gastroenterology,* 2005;11(33): 5180-5184

Coffee Consumption and Risk of Type 2 Diabetes, *Diabetes Care,* February 2014; 37(2);569-586.

Dairy intake is associated with brain glutathione concentration in older adults, *American Journal of Clinical Nutrition,* 2015 101: 287-293.

DASH: Dietary Approaches to Stop Hypertension, http://www.nhlbi.nih.gov/health/public/heart/hbp/dash/new_dash.pdf.

Diabetes Prevention Program, http://www.cdc.gov/diabetes/prevention/about.htm

Dietary fiber, http://www.bmj.com/content/347/bmj.f6879

Dietary Guidelines for Americans, 2010, www.health.gov/dietaryguideline/dga2010/dietaryguidelines2010.pdf

Dietary patterns and colorectal cancer: Systematic review and meta-analysis. *European Journal of Cancer Prevention, 2012;* 21:15–23, 2012.

Examining the health effects of Fructose, David S. Ludwig, MD, PhD, *Journal of the American Medical Asssociation*. 2013;310(1):33-34, http://jama.jamanetwork.com/article.aspx?articleID=1693739

Food and Nutrition for Older Adults: Promoting Health and Wellness," 2012. Position of the Academy of Nutrition and Dietetics

Food, Nutrition, Physical Activity, and the Prevention of Cancer: A Global Perspective, 2007, American Institute for Cancer Research, Washington, DC).

Gatorade Sports Science Institute, http://www.gssiweb.org/about

Gut microbes, *Science*. 2013 Sept 6;341(6150):1241214

Influence of red wine polyphenols and ethanol on the gut microbiota ecology, Maria Queipo-Ortuno et al, *American Journal of Clinical Nutrition, 2012; 95: 1323-1334.*

International Tree Nut Council, www.nuthealth.org

Mediterranean Diet, http://annals.org/article.aspx?articleid=1763229

Milk thistle, http://www.cancer.gov/cancertopics/pdq/cam/milkthistle/Patient/page2

Myth-busting: Butter versus Margarine, Heart Foundation of New Zealand, www.heartfoundation.org.nz/healthy-living/healthy-eating/food-for-a-healthy-heart/replace-butter/myth-busting-butter-versus-margarine

National Cancer Institute, US National Institutes of Health www.cancer.gov

National Center for Alternative and Complementary Medicine (NCCAM) http://nccam.nih.gov.

National Institutes of Health, Office of Dietary Supplements, http://ods.od.nih.gov/factsheets/list-all

National Weight Control Registry, http://www.nwcr.ws/default.htm

New Mexico Chile Pepper Institute, http://www.chilepepperinstitute.org/

Omega-3 and prostate cancer risk, *Journal of the National Cancer Institute*, 2013, http://jnci.oxfordjournals.org/content/early/2013/07/09/jnci.djt174.abstract

Pregnancy weight gain chart, www.iom.edu/About-IOM/Making-a-Difference/Kellogg/~/media/Files/About%20the%20IOM/Pregnancy-Weight/Pregnancyweightzcard.pdf

Produce for Better Health Foundation, http://www.pbhfoundation.org/media/press_rel/pressrelease.php?recordid=486

Spices, www.mccormickspiceinstitute.com

Timing of food intake predicts weight loss effectiveness. *International Journal of Obesity*, 2013;37:624-624.

Vitamin C status and fat oxidation, Carol S. Johnson et al, *Nutrition & Metabolism*, 2006, **3**:35 http://www.nutritionandmetabolism.com/content/3/1/35

Wheat Belly—An Analysis of Selected Statements and Basic Theses from the Book, Julie Jones, PhD, *Cereal World*, July-August 2012, 57 (4), 177-189.

Whey protein, *American Journal of Clinical Nutrition, May 2011, 93 (5): 997-1005; January 2104, 99: 86-95; February 2015, 101 (2): 279-286.*

World Alzheimer Report 2014, <u>http://www.alz.co.uk/research/ WorldAlzheimerReport2014.pdf.</u>

ABOUT THE AUTHOR

Barbara Quinn is a registered dietitian nutritionist (RDN) and certified diabetes educator (CDE) at the Community Hospital of the Monterey Peninsula. Her weekly column QUINN ON NUTRITION appears in the Monterey County Herald and is distributed to media markets worldwide. Quinn lives in Carmel Valley, California.

Made in the USA
San Bernardino, CA
10 December 2017